Animal, Vegetable,

or Woman?

Dearest Jerry,

I hope you enjoy this book
and that it does not put
your life into turmoil -
(I do a little bit actually)

all my love,

Greg

24/5/07

ANIMAL, VEGETABLE, OR WOMAN?

A Feminist Critique
of Ethical Vegetarianism

KATHRYN PAXTON GEORGE

STATE UNIVERSITY OF NEW YORK PRESS

Permission to reprint portions of letters from Deane Curtin to the author, and from Carol J. Adams to the author, are gratefully acknowledged.

Excerpts *passim* from "Discrimination and Bias in the Vegan Ideal," *Journal of Agricultural and Environmental Ethics* 7:1 (1994): 41–76, by Kathryn Paxton George; © 1994; "Use and Abuse Revisited: Response to Pluhar and Varner," *Journal of Agricultural and Environmental Ethics* 7:1 (1994): 41–76, by Kathryn Paxton George; © 1994; "The Use and Abuse of Scientific Studies," *Journal of Agricultural and Enviornmental Ethics* 5:2 (1992): 217–33, by Kathryn Paxton George; © 1992; "So Animal a Human . . . , or the Moral Relevance of Being an Omnivore," *Journal of Agricultural Ethics* 3:2 (Fall 1990): 172–86, by Kathryn Paxton George; © 1990, reprinted with kind permission from Kluwer Academic Publishers.

Excerpts from "Food for Thought," *Religion* 9 (1979), by Julia Twigg; © 1979 reprinted with kind permission of Kluwer Academic Publishers.

Excerpts from "Should Feminists Be Vegetarians?" *Signs: Journal of Women in Culture and Society* 19:2 (Winter 1994): 405–34, by Kathryn Paxton George, © 1994 by The University of Chicago. All rights reserved.

Excerpts from "Reply to Adams, Donovan, Gruen and Gaard," *Signs: Journal of Women in Culture and Society* 21:1 (Autumn 1995): 242–60, by Kathryn Paxton George, © 1995 by The University of Chicago. All rights reserved.

Published by
STATE UNIVERSITY OF NEW YORK PRESS, ALBANY

© 2000 State University of New York

Printed in the United States of America

For information, address State University of New York Press,
90 State Street, Suite 700, Albany, NY 12207

Production, Laurie Searl
Marketing, Anne M. Valentine

Library of Congress Cataloging-in-Publication Data

George, Kathryn Paxton.
    Animal, vegetable, or woman? : a feminist critique of ethical vegetarianism / by Kathryn Paxton George.
        p. cm.
    Includes bibliographical references and index.
    ISBN 0-7914-4687-5 (alk. paper) — ISBN 0-7914-4688-3 (pbk. : alk. paper)
    1. Vegetarianism. 2. Vegetarianism—Moral and ethical aspects. I. Title.

TX392.G46 2000
613.2'62—dc21
                                                                                        99-088561

10   9   8   7   6   5   4   3   2   1

For Bette, Lois, Mickey, Geneva,

Marie, Marian,

Linda,

Sherry, Nancy,

Kim and Francey

CONTENTS

PREFACE

A few years ago, I read Tom Regan's *Case for Animal Rights* (1983). His arguments convinced me to become a vegetarian, and I was able to convince my husband to adopt this diet as well. But I was less sure about whether my ten-year-old daughter should adopt it. I was especially concerned about whether to omit milk from her diet. At about the same time, a nutrition colleague asked me to team-teach a course on animal rights. In the unit on ethical vegetarianism, he presented basic nutritional information that vegan and vegetarian diets are safe when well-planned. But he expressed concerns about vegan diets for infants, children, adolescents, and pregnant and lactating women because their needs were increased for several kinds of nutrients. Vegans omit all meat, fish, and animal products such as milk and eggs from their diets. In contrast, most vegetarians include milk, eggs, and sometimes fish and chicken (Dwyer 1993b).

Because of my scientific background, I felt capable of researching the nutrition studies myself. Aware of how often the mass media distorts information about nutrition, I sought out original research sources and I discussed my readings with several nutritionists and scientists. Over the last several years, I have come to see the deep male biases of the traditional arguments for ethical vegetarianism. While it is touted as an ideal lifestyle, ethical vegetarianism actually discriminates against women, infants, children, adolescents, some of the elderly, nonwhite races and ethnicities, and those living in cultures that are not westernized or industrialized. In this book, I explain in detail why choosing a vegetarian diet for the sake of animals or a feminist ideal is much more complicated than many ethical vegetarians might have expected. I explain why, even though my husband and I chose vegetarian diets, I could not restrict my daughter's diet, nor would I claim that anyone has a *moral* requirement to choose vegetarianism or to regard it as a moral ideal. Yet, there remain other reasons for some people to choose vegetarianism, such as for health or preference. Nothing in what is said here should be interpreted to mean that vegan or vegetarian diets are unhealthy or dangerous in the proper settings. It is one thing to choose a vegetarian diet for reasons of health or preference and quite another to praise it as a moral ideal or to make it a moral requirement.

A fair amount of nutritional research literature is presented in this book, not only to support my argument but also to inform readers who may be current vegetarians or are considering this diet. To the best of my ability, I present what I found to be the "all things considered" judgment of nutritionists based on experimental research, as given in textbooks, reviews, and special issues of journals with high standards of scholarship. To get the reference list, I did computer and library searches to learn both sides of these questions. Unless noted in the references, when I have cited a source, I have read the entire article. I present what I found, not to argue that there is no controversy, but to show that there are *undisputed differences* in the nutritional requirements among women, men, children, the old, and those in other cultures. Many of these nutritional differences indicate physiological differences that are reflected in the Recommended Daily Allowances (RDAs) published by the National Research Council (1989b), but I do not expect readers to see my point from mere citation of the RDAs. In some instances, the information presented reflects research that was used in setting the most recent RDAs.

The change to a vegetarian diet happened to be easy for me. I have little attachment to any particular food. Even my husband gave up meat rather easily. But I do care about doing the right thing, and I attribute the ease of my change-over to the appeal of the moral rights arguments of Tom Regan and Bernard Rollin and, to a lesser extent, Peter Singer. At one time, the rights position seemed more logically and practically consistent to me, and utilitarian arguments do not seem to meet that criterion. For several years I remained convinced that I was living as morally as possible with respect to animals, even though I did not take up the vegan way and I did not believe I should try to convert my daughter to a vegetarian diet. From my research, she, at least, would have no obligation to follow a vegetarian diet.

At the time I began the reading, I was teaching courses in the rights and welfare of animals and veterinary ethics; I also included a section on the morality of using animals in medical research in my medical ethics courses. It was not until the spring of 1991 that I realized the inherent male bias in these arguments. The occasion occurred in listening to a paper being given by Gary Varner, a philosopher from Texas A & M University, on why dairy products are immoral. Suddenly, and surprisingly, I became incensed—Gary will probably not forget this—as I realized that women, children, and others were being forgotten in the argument for the "vegan ideal" as the most virtuous diet. I immediately wrote a short paper and circulated it to philosophical friends. At the same time I resumed my nutrition research to obtain greater detail. My colleague, Janice Capel Anderson, also from University of Idaho, read my paper and started me in the direction of feminist alternatives in ethical theory. More than anyone, Jan has contributed to helping me plumb the depths of my feminist concerns. For that I am deeply grateful.

In the "Preface" to the second edition of *Animal Liberation* (1990), Peter Singer comments on the way the animal liberation movement has grown since the first edition was published in 1975. He remarks that all of the activists are now vegetarian and that even conservatives are apologetic about serving meat and usually offer alternatives. Singer admits that "in my dreams, at least, everyone who read the book was going to say, 'Yes, of course . . . ,' and would immediately become vegetarian and start protesting against what we do to animals" (1990, ix). That's how it was for me. Perhaps I have convinced some students to become vegetarians; I know that many were convinced by the rights and utilitarian arguments we read in class. There is irony in the fact that I now believe that these arguments serve the ruling, patriarchal class. Should I dream that people will read this book and discover the bias and come to care not simply about animals but also about women, children, the elderly, and people in other cultures? I hope they will and that they will reconsider their reasons for being vegetarians.

ACKNOWLEDGMENTS

Thanks are due to the many colleagues who have read, critiqued, and shared information and ideas for this book. Among them are Jeffrey Burkhardt, Leo K. Bustad, Gary Comstock, Deane Curtin, Nicholas Gier, Marvin Henberg, Harry O. Kunkel, Bernard E. Rollin, Carolyn Sachs, Deborah Smith, Paul B. Thompson, and Karen Warren. Thanks also to Carol Adams, Josephine Donovan, Greta Gaard and Lori Gruen, as well as Evelyn Pluhar and Gary Varner for their incisive criticisms. I am especially grateful to Alison Jaggar for her willingness to discuss the original paper with me and for the useful suggestions she made about counterarguments. John Froseth and Val Hillers have served as nutrition advisors, although the research is my own. As noted above, my colleague Janice Capel Anderson has contributed much to further my understanding of issues in feminism. Thanks so much to Shelley Hill, my research assistant, for tracking down so many articles for me; also Lorel Getty, Jeff Marks, Judey Nitcy, and Topher Taylor for proofreading and checking references. A shorter version of the argument of this book was published earlier in *Signs* (George 1994b), and the editors and reviewers were an immense help in providing constructive criticism and assistance; special thanks to Kate Tyler, who was then a member of the *Signs* editorial staff. I would also like to thank the SUNY Press reviewers and editors. The research was supported in part by grants from the University of Idaho Research Council, the Idaho State Board of Education, and the National Science Foundation. The opinions expressed herein are my own and not necessarily those of the National Science Foundation, the State of Idaho, or the University of Idaho. I would also like to thank the University of Idaho for a sabbatical leave during which I completed the first draft of this book.

CHAPTER 1

INTRODUCTION

VEGETARIANISM AND THE IDEAL LIFE

In his book, *Rachel and Her Children*, Jonathan Kozol (1988) interviews some of the poor and homeless of New York City. Mr. Alessandro, an Italian American man, has lost his wife, his job, his home, and 45 pounds from hunger. He lives with his 73-year-old mother and his three children in a single room in the Martinique Hotel (54–59). Every day Mr. Alessandro looks for work and he looks for permanent housing on a welfare allowance too small ever to give him hope of leaving the hotel. His food stamp allowance for himself and the three children is $50 per month (60). During the interview Kozol realizes that the children are quite literally starving. He gives Mr. Alessandro $20 to buy food. There is no local supermarket, only a convenience store. Mr. Alessandro brings back "a box of Kellogg's Special K, a gallon of juice, a half-gallon of milk, a loaf of bread, a dozen eggs, a package of sausages, a roll of toilet paper" (59). Rachel and her children live in the same hotel in a similar room:

> When we moved here I was forced to sign a paper. Everybody has to do it. It's a promise that you will not cook inside your room. So we lived on cold bologna (66).
> Plenty of children livin' here on nothin' but bread and bologna. Peanut butter. Jelly. Drinkin' water. You buy milk. I bought one gallon yesterday. Got *this* much left. They drink it fast. Orange juice, they drink it fast. End up drinkin' Kool Aid (68).

1

These are America's urban poor. In 1987 in New York City alone, 700,000 of them were children (5). Most of these children live in households headed by women. They do not have a healthy diet. Their parents cannot cook fresh vegetables for them, even if they could buy them. Although many hotel residents break the rules and use hotplates, Kozol attests to the difficulty of cooking any kind of meal in these conditions. Many hotel residents do not even have refrigerators to keep food from spoiling.

Does Rachel do something wrong when she buys bologna and milk for her children to eat? Some philosophers and some feminists who argue for ethical vegetarianism based on the moral equality of animals would say yes. But, of course, most would agree that Rachel is to be excused. She cannot help doing such a wrongful act because her circumstances force her to it. We aren't supposed to blame her but forgive her.

Penny is an anemic pregnant American woman who has been faithfully taking her iron supplements while following a vegetarian diet. Her obstetrician advises that she should have a blood transfusion to bring up her hemoglobin (blood iron) level. Alternatively, she could try eating beef liver two or three times a week. She could do neither and forget about the anemia. What should she choose? If she chooses to eat liver after assessing the risks of contracting hepatitis or other blood-borne diseases, has she done something wrong?

Probably most moralists would leave the decision up to her, and even those arguing for the equal rights of animals would probably excuse her for choosing to try eating the liver. Circumstance and physiology make Penny and Rachel unable to live up to the ideal proposed by ethical vegetarianism—to live without killing animals or causing them any suffering. Many who strive to live as ethical vegetarians adopt the vegan diet and lifestyle, using no flesh, eggs, milk, or other animal products. This is the "vegan ideal" and those who adopt it on moral grounds believe that it is the best, most virtuous way to live (cf. Singer 1975, 181). Unfortunately, Penny, Rachel, Mr. Alessandro, his aging mother, and their children cannot live that way—yet. Part of the politics of the vegan ideal is that it should be possible for all people to adopt this lifestyle. Is this a worthy goal? If you believe, as I do, that the sufferings of animals are as morally important as those of humans, how can we not think so?

This book questions the vegan ideal and the goals of ethical vegetarianism by exposing unstated assumptions in the moral arguments for that position. I will argue that the ideal itself is discriminatory because a single definable class of persons is designated as better than—more *morally virtuous* than—all others simply because of its physiology and its power. I challenge all four major defenses of the claim that most humans ought to be vegetarians because animals have moral standing. Each of these views elevates and morally idealizes the vegan lifestyle as most virtuous, although to varying degrees. All four defenses contain a hidden assumption that having an adult male body and living in cultures where adequate food and supplementation are available are the norm. Those who present these defenses—Tom Regan, Peter Singer, Carol Adams, and Deane Curtin, in particular—falsely (and probably unwittingly) assume that there is no significant difference in the nutritional needs of males and females and children and the elderly. In order to make their moral arguments, these scholars must rely on conclusions drawn from nutritional studies done on adult males in industrialized countries. In addition, the scholars must ignore or dismiss studies and epidemiological evidence of the shortcomings of such diets for other age groups and for many women. I call this skewed assumption the "male physiological ideal." The ideal pervades both nutritional science and moral argument: women, children, and others are referred to in the scientific literature as "nutritionally vulnerable" with respect to certain vitamins and minerals such as iron, calcium, vitamin D, and zinc. All current arguments for ethical vegetarianism treat such "nutritional vulnerability" as an *exception* rather than as a norm. The norm is defined by the adult male body, which is less "vulnerable" to the adverse health consequences of vegetarian diets. But, the very fact that the majority lives as a mere exception suggests that the ideal is skewed in favor of a group in power. The hidden assumption in the moral arguments is that *being less vulnerable is good,* simply because one is *stronger,* and *being vulnerable is bad* or, at least not as good, because one is *weaker.* But that is a bald argument for power rather than for justice, moral virtue, or caring. In the examination of each of the four defenses, I attempt to show that both the traditional moral theoretical ethics and current feminist contextualist ethics fail on grounds of arbitrariness; that is, the mere imposition of power through acceptance of a false belief. The false belief is that the adult male body is, for practical nutritional purposes, the same as that of the adult female, the adolescent, the child, or the elderly. It fails to recognize material differences among humans. If they wish to act rightly and yet accept this false belief, women, adolescents, children, the elderly, and others would be forced to suffer greater burdens than men, disadvantaging these groups with respect to health and economic power. If people in lower economic classes and nonindustrialized cultures accept this false belief and the attendant moral arguments, they will count it as morally obligatory to live in a way that is most compatible for adult males (age 20–50) living in industrialized societies. Thus, the power enjoyed by the most powerful will be perpetuated. I argue that this, in turn, perpetuates an unjust belief (or suspicion) that women and those who are less well off economically are *morally* weaker because they are *physically* weaker or live in circumstances without an industrialized food system. Thus, morality becomes a club used for power rather than for justice. A truly virtuous person should be defined by his or her choices, acts, and moral character and not by her or his physical make-up.

The "vegan ideal," as I am referring to it here, is a vision of human beings or the world to which some persons think we should all aspire. Those who endorse it currently believe it is a moral ideal, rather than a nonmoral, psychological, or aesthetic ideal. Continuous practice in the attempt to attain the vegan ideal results in possession of a character trait or a virtue that would be considered morally good in any human being regardless of gender, age, or ethnicity. The attitude may be similar to that seen in religious history; the most virtuous persons were regarded as saints. In Western society, many of our secular ethical ideals have their origins in religion. Ancient Greek and Stoic ethics were commingled with Judeo-Christian-Islamic dogma in late Roman and Medieval times (Jones 1969). The vision of the vegan or vegetarian life as most perfect arises from complex religious, cultural, and agricultural practices that we will not be able to explore in this book. But it is worth noting that all major world religions have vegetarian sects within them. Restrictions on meat consumption are often thought to improve the soul and promote rationalistic and mystical knowledge. Christian saints, both male and female, were revered for their ability to survive on a limited diet of bread (usually the host) and water—a vegan ideal (Bell 1985; Bynum 1987). In fact, bread and wine (both all-plant foods) are still the celebrated Christian sacred symbols of life and spirit. The idealization of food practice is associated with class distinctions and the search for hierarchical power. It separates "real" men from other men, women from men, the poor from the rich, the "dregs" of society from the "highest and most holy."

The Western or Eurocentric concept of animal rights and the drive to place the lives and sufferings of animals on an equal footing with that of humans arises from a moral tradition spanning more than two millennia. This tradition began with the moral teachings of the ancient Greeks and continued through the Enlightenment and into the present day. After the French and American Revolutions, morality became more secularized in the Western world. Human beings envisioned a society where individuals could be free to worship as they chose, and philosophers such as Immanuel Kant in Prussia and Jeremy Bentham and John Stuart Mill in England developed secular ethical theories that were meant to bridge the common moral ground shared by all human beings. The utilitarians Bentham and Mill wished to set aside all "intuitive" moral rules and political restrictions unless such rules could be shown to cause more good than suffering or harm. From the political writings of Thomas Hobbes, John Locke, and others, as well as from Kant's duty-based moral theory, the idea of human rights arose. Rights gained popular appeal because they afforded protections for ordinary people against the oppressive power of the state and society. Governmental leaders could no longer rule by fiat or by inheritance but were held accountable to the people. The vision of a community of equals—of fraternity (but, alas, not yet of sorority)—gripped the imaginations of leaders who lived then and of many who live now. The rights of the powerless and vulnerable would thereafter cry to be respected. In the last years of the eighteenth century and throughout of nineteenth, feminists such as Mary Wollstonecraft argued for the rights of women, abolitionists such as William Lloyd Garrison and Sarah and Angelina Grimké argued against slavery, and anti-vivisectionists such as Henry Salt and Frances Power Cobbe argued for the rights of animals.[1]

Today, Tom Regan (1983) and Peter Singer (1975, 1981) use the traditional secular moral theories developed in the Kantian and utilitarian traditions, respectively. Animals can suffer and be "subjects-of-a-life" and so must be counted as members of the moral community. As a practical outcome, both argue explicitly for a rule of moral vegetarianism. People who follow the rule are moral; those who do not are immoral. By direct implication, persons who *consistently* follow such rules are said to be virtuous; those who ignore or fail to obey valid moral rules are said to be vicious.[2] Following rules requires people to make choices and to act in accordance with their moral beliefs. In that way, people are judged for what they do rather than on the basis of their sex, race, or class.

If Regan and Singer are correct, virtuous people would be vegetarians at least, and vegans ideally because veganism is said to respect life and incur the least animal suffering. Regan and Singer both endorse the "vegan ideal."[3] In their view, attempting to realize the ideal is *morally required* of good people. A good person does not choose veganism as a simple act of kindness toward animals, because charity is not required in any strong sense. On their view *justice* requires the pursuit of the vegan ideal. Following a simple moral rule forbidding the killing of nonthreatening animals is required for all truly good people—people of integrity, virtue, and high moral character—people who wish to be charitable *and* just.

Many feminists have joined Regan and Singer in efforts to awaken people to moral concern for animals. Carol Adams (1990, 1991, 1993, 1994), Josephine Donovan (1990), Greta Gaard (1993), Marti Kheel (1985) and many others have championed the rights of animals as essential to feminism. For these writers and others, the vegan ideal is a feminist ideal.[4] Ideals underlie many of our psychological motivations, and history and culture can be changed by the ideals we adopt. So, having the right ideals and knowing why we believe them to be right is extremely important.

Writers in feminist ethics question rule-centered, rationalistic traditional moral theory and its psychology of moral development, arguing that these serve to legitimate the actions of the class in power—largely white males. For example, Carol Gilligan (1982) argues that women experience a different moral development. Gilligan claims that women prefer a moral language of care, responsibilities, and relationships among people, whereas males usually prefer to speak a language of rules, rights, and justice. Other feminists such as Virginia Held (1987, 1993, 1995) and Sara Ruddick (1989) argue for caring, empathy, and maternal thinking as ways of knowing and foundations for feminist ethical thought. Nel Noddings (1984) focuses on caring as a relational experience to build a unique *feminine* (versus feminist) ethics. In fact, each feminist thinker has added her or his own particular ideas to the nascent field of feminist ethics. Virtually all of these thinkers reject the traditional rights and utilitarian theoretical approaches, however (Tong 1993). Why so? Rights are explicated in terms of interests that are supposedly common to all persons and so are impersonal and universal, rather than particular and contextual. Feminists usually object that interests are too abstract. Focussing on interests instead of people and their relationships tends to decontextualize moral problems. Traditional moral theories such as rights or utilitarianism tend to view individuals in isolation or as "atoms" rather than people in relation. In most cases they also emphasize the ascendancy of reason over empathy, sentiment, or emotion in knowing right from wrong.[5] Such rationalistic arguments center on justification of universal rules and on justifications for exceptions to them with primary attention given to the demands of the individual. Some feminists argue that, at their worst, these moral justifications become a part of civil and criminal law, which then become a club that may be held over the vulnerable, to ignore, attack, or destroy relationship rather than to uphold it (Littleton 1987; MacKinnon 1985, 1989). The contemporary feminists discussed here and later would agree that all moral decision making must be judged in concrete context and with respect to relationships rather than in abstraction as if individuals act in isolation.

The foregoing gives you a brief outline of the history and rationale for adopting ethical vegetarianism. Now think about the situations and contexts of Rachel and Penny. Is it merely their environments that disadvantage them? I will argue that their "context" involves being female, being mothers, and that they do not need to be excused or forgiven for not being vegetarians. Instead, we need to rethink the ideal assumed in ethical vegetarianism.

In the next section I discuss the various meanings of "vegetarianism," and in the following section, I explain what I will cover in the book and what I will leave out. Finally, I give an overview of the main arguments of this book.

A NOTE ABOUT TERMS AND STUDIES OF VEGETARIANS

One important element of being ethical is being consistent in our beliefs and our decision making. Although no two situations are exactly alike, often enough resemblance exists across cases that we can say it would be wrong to treat them differently. If scientists and ethicists are to have an adequate understanding of nutrition, then, they need consistent criteria for deciding whom to call a vegetarian and whom to call an omnivore. Without these criteria, the data would become confounded and meaningless. The same is true of trying to do the right thing. Although we cannot expect to be perfect or obtain "laboratory conditions" in comparing contexts, we need to adopt the same meanings of the words we use and try to develop some understanding of the kinds of factors that will or will not count in making a defensible decision. For example, it is defensible to hire the person with the best skills but indefensible to hire a person with no skills applicable to a job simply because the boss "takes a shine" to him or her, and we shouldn't change the meaning of "skills" from one person to the next. So, in our case about vegetarianism, we need to know what counts as a vegetarian. Those arguing for ethical vegetarianism suppose that vegetarian diets are healthy for virtually all persons, which is a claim that relies on modern nutritional research for its accuracy. Therefore, those making ethical arguments should adopt the same definitions that nutritional scientists used in conducting their health studies. Below I define the meanings of various "vegetarianisms" by quoting the definitions used by nutritional researchers. I also compare these with the common usages found by social scientists.

In everyday language, the term "vegetarian" is used with a great deal of variation, whereas "vegan" has a more precise meaning for food practice. A vegan eats no fish or animal flesh and avoids milk, eggs, and other animal products as well; sometimes vegans are referred to as "strict vegetarians." Beardsworth and Keil (1991) did a sociological study of people in the United Kingdom who defined themselves as "vegetarians," and they found that some people who occasionally eat meat (as well as fish and animal products) may define themselves as "vegetarian"—about five percent did so. Another twenty-five percent ate fish, eggs, and dairy products; thirty-four percent, "lactoovovegetarians," omitted the fish; twelve percent were "lactovegetarians," omitting all animal flesh and products except dairy; the remaining twenty-four percent were vegans.

Such self-definitions would not lend themselves well to the scientific study of the nutritional consequences of vegetarianism. Researchers need to establish a standard against which to judge the content of a diet that is given a particular name. They also need to know what people are actually eating in order to gauge the adequacy of the diet. In citing nutrition literature and using the term "vegetarian" and "vegan," my intention is to match as closely as possible the categories experimental researchers have used for their subjects in determination of results. Johanna T. Dwyer, a world authority on vegetarian diets, especially in children, has done extensive research and publication in this area (Dwyer *et al.* 1978, 1980; Jacobs and Dwyer 1988; Dwyer 1988; Dwyer 1991; Dwyer 1993a,b; Dwyer and Loew 1994, among others). In "Vegetarianism in Children" (1993b), Dwyer gives the following definitions:

> Vegans, or total vegetarians, consume no animal products. This is the rarest form of vegetarianism. . . . Lactovegetarian diets include plant foods, milk, and dairy products, but they exclude all meat, fish, poultry, and eggs. This type of vegetarianism is relatively rare (174).

Lactoovovegetarian diets add eggs to the lactovegetarian diet and are the most common form of vegetarianism. Dwyer (1993b) continues:

> Semivegetarian diets include plant foods, milk and dairy products, eggs, and some fish and poultry. They are increasingly common, probably more so than any other form of vegetarianism, especially among young adults. Although many vegetarians do not believe that semivegetarian diets are truly vegetarian, those who eat them regard themselves as vegetarians. Red meat is avoided or eaten only occasionally, and other forms of flesh may also be limited or eaten only in small amounts (175).

When I use the term "vegetarians," I will generally be referring to "lactoovovegetarians." When I use the term "vegan," I refer to those who eat virtually no animal flesh or product (or so little that nutritionists consider the nutrient contribution to be nil). "Semivegetarian diets," where used in my own arguments, refers to the above definition and would not exclude small amounts of red meat.

These usages do not define exact eating patterns. Even within the vegan or largely vegan lifestyle, variation occurs in the eating pattern due to the reasons people have for adopting veganism. Jacobs and Dwyer (1988) report different nutritional intakes for children in the vegan religious groups: Black Hebrews, Zen macrobiotics, and Rastifarians. Perhaps the largest group of lactoovovegetarians in the world are Hindus, and perhaps the most studied group are Seventh-Day Adventists in the United States. "New" vegetarians in the United States are people who have adopted vegan or vegetarian diets as adults for philosophical, ecological, religious, or health reasons. Several studies were done on "new" vegetarians in the late 1970s and early 1980s. The animal rights and welfare movements have precipitated new conversions to vegetarian and vegan diets. In Western countries, few people adopt vegetarian or vegan diets for economic reasons (Dwyer 1991, 1993a,b), but in developing nations many people are often vegetarians of necessity (Dwyer and Loew 1994). Foods of animal origin are not present, and the variety of plant foods that people can get is limited. Anemias and deficiencies are common in many areas of the Third World[6] (Scrimshaw 1991). The simple addition of meat to the diets of people in "obligatory vegan" cultures would not solve their nutritional problems—a balance of foods is always needed that emphasizes grains, legumes, fruits, and vegetables. But they often need food of any kind and moralizing about meat eating in other cultures is inconsistent with feminism.

Several kinds of studies have been done on those living in vegetarian cultures, such as Hindus, and on established and "new" vegetarians in Western countries. In each case, the researcher takes a profile of what the patient or subject actually eats. There are, generally, six kinds of reports seen in the literature: (1) clinical reports of people who have presented themselves to a doctor or hospital with a dietary deficiency (often these are women, infants, children, or elderly people); (2) reviews of relevant scientific studies of vegans or vegetarians; (3) retrospective studies in which a group of people (often very large) with and without a particular disease condition is asked to recall a dietary pattern to correlate specific nutrients with a disease or deficiency; (4) prospective studies in which normal people (controls and study group) are asked to give a profile of their diet, blood, urine and other samples or tests, and are followed to see whether disease processes related to diet develop; (5) "blind" and (6) "double-blind"[7] studies in which an experimental group and a control group eat a specified diet and are then monitored and tested for specific results, such as blood pressure, calcium loss, and so forth.

Health benefits are well-documented for some kinds of American and European vegetarian lifestyles: "Data are strong that vegetarians are at lesser risk for obesity, atonic constipation, lung cancer, and alcoholism. Evidence is good that risks for hypertension, coronary artery disease, type II diabetes, and gallstones are lower" (Dwyer 1988, 712).[8] Vegetarians who have been studied always adopt a set of practices in addition to diet that affects health risks and out-comes. The vegetarians most often studied usually limit or omit tobacco, caf-feine, and alcohol. Often they are very health-conscious and include physical exercise in their lives. Very often, religious and spiritual beliefs are associated with vegetarianism. Yet, the data on relative benefits for adult males versus females and children that can reliably be ascribed to diet are mixed, with bene-fits in some cases favoring adult males. Some studies of vegetarian males appear to show benefits; some studies and reports on vegetarian and especially vegan women and children appear to show risks. These facts are documented in detail in chapter 4.

SOME ARGUMENTS NOT COVERED

This book is not intended to argue against all possible moral *reasons* for adopt-ing vegetarianism. Instead, I aim to show that the decision to adopt vegetarian-ism involves contextual judgment that cannot appeal to a general moral rule commanding ethical vegetarianism nor can one command it as a virtue that devolves from a vegan ideal. If one chooses vegetarianism, as I did for several years, it will be from a variety of nonmoral reasons. Instead, I argue for a femi-nist aesthetic semivegetarianism because it is more consistently egalitarian in its consideration of all members of the moral community. And my view will accommodate differences among the species while working toward a functional view of equality. Feminist aesthetic vegetarianism will be quasi-ethical in that it is limited by an egalitarianism that balances a number of values and freedoms simultaneously. These arguments will be developed in chapter 7.

At least four other theory-based arguments are often given that socially conscious people in wealthy countries should be moral vegans or vegetarians.[9] I shall not cover these arguments in depth here, but I will outline them and cri-tique them briefly to distinguish them from the specific arguments that I intend to rebut. First, the *argument against factory farming:* People in wealthy countries eat an excessive amount of meat. This consumption means that huge numbers of animals are raised in "industrialized" conditions of short lives, cramped con-ditions, discomfort, and injury. And regardless of how good farming condi-tions of animals might be, their production is exploitive and/or taking their lives is wrong. Eating any meat at all underwrites these conditions, and a moral person would not participate in these practices. Second, the *argument from public health:* vegan and vegetarian diets have health advantages. Everyone, or most everyone, would be healthier if Americans were converted to these diets. And public policymakers are morally obligated to promote vegetarian diets to minimize public health burdens that occur secondary to meat-consumption. Third, the *argument from global health:* vegetarian and vegan lifestyles are morally required to save the Earth because industrialized animal production is causing continuous environmental degradation such as decimation of rain forests in Central and South America, desertification in Africa, and degradation of publicly owned grazing lands in the American West. Fourth, the *argument from peace and nonviolence:* a good person should be committed to nonviolence and oppose killing whether or not discrimination against some classes of people occurs, and so animals should not be killed for food or any other reason. In the following subsections, I offer brief critiques of each of these arguments. In morality, we should make choices for the *right reasons.* While some of the reasons below are good reasons for many people to avoid meat eating, the first three are utilitarian arguments that do not consider the question of whether killing or using food animals is intrinsically evil or wrongful. The fourth argument considers all killing to be wrongful, but carries with it consequences that most morally good people would not wish to live with.

FACTORY FARMING

Most food animals in countries where meat consumption is high are raised in intensive agricultural housing or so-called "factory farms." Animals may be penned in stalls so small that reclining or turning around is impossible (for example, swine stalls) or in conditions of crowding and darkness never seen in nature (for example, poultry batteries). Although improvements in conditions for farm animals have improved in recent years because of legislation, most animal rights and welfare advocates find confinement agriculture morally objectionable. Extreme confinement is inhumane and that judgment follows from a general proscription against cruelty. Many animal advocates and ethical vegetarians claim that giving up species equality and ethical vegetarianism will mean losing protections for animals and a continuation of cruelty to them. But the proscription against cruelty does not mean that we must grant equality or rights to other species. Even if such animals are not morally equal with humans, humans are still required not to cause them pain, distress, or frustration of their natural needs and behaviors. One need not support the vegan ideal to accomplish the goal of minimizing animal suffering. Free-range eggs and milk from pastured cows are available in some areas, and cattle, sheep, swine, and chickens can be raised humanely. To argue against factory farming, one need not embrace the "either/or" of veganism versus "animal-based" diets and excessive meat.

Abandonment of the vegan or vegetarian moral position would not permit an exacerbation of animal cruelty. The potential for suffering, harm, and mortality remain at the center of moral concern, and humans have always been enjoined by their moral teachers to treat animals with care and respect (Regan 1986).

PUBLIC HEALTH

On this argument, if public health officials promoted vegan or vegetarian diets, the human population would be healthier. In the arena of public policy, considerations of benefits have merit and may bolster utilitarian arguments for the moral value of vegetarian diets even if animals are not counted as equals. Elected representatives and appointed bureaucrats are supposed to act for the good of the populace. Promoting vegan or vegetarian diets certainly might be an improvement over the high-fat, badly balanced omnivorous diets now consumed in the industrialized world. This argument appeals heavily to factual concerns and becomes a moral argument only when coupled with the duty of public officials to promote the public good. Some of the factual claims include: High-fat diets cause poorer health in a substantial portion of the population. Vegetarian diets are lower in fat than omnivorous diets.[10] Value claims include the belief that health is better than disease and that public officials have duties to promote the good for their constituents. The argument is conditional: If public health officials want x (a healthier populace), then they ought to promote y (vegetarian diets). Because health is desirable and public officials must promote the public good, they are required to promote x, and so they must promote y. A substantial portion of this book is devoted to consideration of the facts (see chapter 4). But even if the factual claims were true, several flaws are apparent in the reasoning. For instance, showing that "meat-centered" diets are bad does not show that vegan diets are ideally healthful and environmentally sound. Semivegetarian diets can be quite low in fat for those groups who need such low-fat diets—but children need diets that have dense, higher caloric value. Low-fat diets may not be good for them. Adult men appear to benefit from vegetarian diets more than women and children in trade-offs for cardiac health, osteoporosis, and other risks. Semivegetarian diets are better for general adoption because they are healthful and pose little or no nutritional risk, and I will show that feminist aesthetic semivegetarianism is *fairer* because it is non-discriminatory and serves the values of community and equity better than the vegan ideal.

ENVIRONMENTAL HEALTH

Some ecofeminists (for instance, Adams 1991) and American environmentalists believe that vegetarian and vegan lifestyles are morally required to save the
Earth (Lewis 1994). They often cite Frances Moore Lappé (1971). Industrialized animal production is causing continuous destruction of rain forests in
Central and South America, desertification in Africa, and degradation of publicly owned grazing lands in the American West. Raising too many animals on
land that could be used to raise grain is a "protein factory in reverse" because
cattle consume more protein than they produce. Does *environmental concern*
require vegetarianism? Environmental vegetarians wish to force the industrialized food system to downscale, to reduce or virtually eliminate demand for beef
and other meat whose production results in environmental degradation, and to
reverse some of the political damage that has been done to indigenous cultures
by Western economic exploitation (Gussow 1994).[11] These are pressing problems that need solutions soon. Unfortunately, they cannot be solved or amelio-
rated by eliminating food animal production. Ecofeminists underscore the
need for sustainable food production, but animals are an integral part of all
known sustainable food systems (Gussow 1994).

Crop production is no less industrialized than animal production, both
here and abroad, and many of our fruits and vegetables are imported. Restruc-
turing during "development" in many parts of Latin America, Africa, and Asia
has impoverished many peasants who once fed themselves from their own garden plots. They were forced off the land to make way for large farms that now
grow a single crop (called "monocropping"). Land has been concentrated into
the hands of a few wealthy families, who hire the landless peasants, often at
lower than subsistence wages. Monocropping in areas that once raised a variety
of plants and animals cuts local availability of foods (see Lappé and Collins
1986). In some areas, malnutrition is a constant problem, and workers subsist,
often unsuccessfully, by trying to take large amounts of vitamin supplements.
These farming methods are unsustainable, exhaust the soil and resources, and
impoverish whole classes of people. Women are often disproportionately bur-
dened and disenfranchised (Shiva 1989).

A more sustainable, regenerative crop production is needed, and some cultures have sustained such systems for thousands of years. Joan Dye Gussow
(1994) notes that these sustainable farming systems depend heavily on the integration of livestock with crops (see also Shiva 1989). In her tenth edition of
Diet for a Small Planet, Lappé (1982) underscores this fact and argues for

reduced consumption but not abolition of animal production. Environmentalists will want to study the interrelation of domestic species, both plant and animal, with an open mind and avoid preconceived notions that food animal production is intrinsically bad and something to be "overcome" in a biocentrically organized, humane world.

PACIFISM AND NONVIOLENCE

Vegetarianism has been connected to peacefulness, and many feminist writers claim nonviolence as the highest stage of feminist ethical life (Gilligan 1977, 1982; Ruddick 1989; and others). Deane Curtin connects his contextual moral vegetarianism with nonviolence, but stops short of pacifism. Pacifism differs from a principle of nonviolence or peacefulness. A pacifist abjures killing in all forms virtually without exception. Although I know of no feminist vegetarian making such a radically pacifist claim, both the feminist and the traditionalist could justify ethical vegetarianism on pacifist grounds as a fallback position in the face of my arguments in this book. The tenet may be stated as follows: Even if some classes and cultures, women, infants, and old people would be discriminated against, the right of an animal to its own life is sacrosanct and linked to the important value of nonviolence. Even if the health of some humans is adversely affected, exceptions do not hold, and killing an animal for food or other uses is always wrong.

The traditional pacifist position has some plausible defenses that I shall not be able to discuss here. But the position is utterly self-sacrificial and is the only position consistent with according strict equality to the worth of animal lives. It appears to fit best into stage two of Gilligan's moral development scheme (1982). In that stage, a caring person (usually a woman) chooses from the "good of self-sacrifice." At the higher stage three, the caring person comes to see that she herself has value and that no one should be sacrificed or hurt. According to feminists of this bent (but not all feminists by any stretch), this realization propels the person to an ideal of nonviolence.

I find the pacifist position untenable because the position can require parents to sacrifice the needs of their children in important circumstances. Also, the moral burden of being a pacifist will fall more heavily on parents than on the childless, for parents form bonds of responsibility for the child which cannot in good conscience be forsaken or forgotten at the moment of choice between the life of an animal and the health or life of their children. Like other absolutisms, pacifism will fail to recognize the nuances of context and circumstance. Pacifism requires subsuming the duties of caring and protecting one's child to an absolute prohibition on killing.

Self-sacrificial pacifism also undermines morality—it takes away an important reason we have for living morally in the first place. Among the usual rejoinders offered against being immoral is that each individual will benefit by living in a society where everyone follows moral rules or is relatively virtuous and responsible. If following those rules or adopting a virtue would require that you give up your life or sacrifice your child, then pure egoism or "immorality" is likely to be more persuasive. A self-sacrificial pacifism that discriminates against vulnerable classes of people and favors the strong seems particularly noxious because it follows a pattern of instituting moral codes that favor the privileged class, giving the illusion that others are "naturally immoral."

OVERVIEW OF THE ARGUMENT OF THE BOOK

The book presents an original argument challenging all the current arguments for ethical vegetarianism based on the rights or welfare of animals. I show that neither traditional moral theory nor current feminist ethics will sustain a moral command to ethical vegetarianism. From within moral rights theory and utilitarianism, the arguments for the interests of animals are plausible, and a rule of ethical vegetarianism appears to follow from accepting the tenets of either theory. But, I argue that such arguments are ultimately unsuccessful because they violate their own more central principles of universality, impartiality, and equality. This means that a moral rule requiring ethical vegetarianism discriminates against women, children, older persons, and those in nonindustrial or nonwesternized cultural settings. The vegan ideal also entrenches patriarchy.

Traditional moral theory relies on the Principle of Equality of all people, regardless of race, sex, age, or class. Although males and females differ in some respects, they share the attribute of being mortal and capacities for pain, unhappiness, happiness, and self-fulfillment. Arguments for the equality of nonhuman animals "expand the circle" of moral concern to other species. Peter Singer used the analogy of racism or sexism to condemn speciesism—the exclusion of animals from the domain of equality. But my argument shows that, if we believe that sexism is wrong, then we must *accept* speciesism—animals cannot be the equals of humans. But if we *reject* speciesism, then we must accept sexism and the belief that women cannot be the equal of men. This will mean that traditional moral arguments for the rights and welfare of animals are logically inconsistent and collapse on their own foundations. That being so, these traditional moral arguments for ethical vegetarianism cannot be integrated into a feminist ethic.

Moreover, specifically feminist arguments for ethical vegetarianism or the vegan ideal must also fail: the vegan ideal cannot be a feminist ideal. Although some feminists believe that any adequate feminist ethic must reject consuming meat and animal products, I will show that even the feminist arguments assume a male norm to which women are expected to accommodate themselves unfairly. Briefly, anyone committed to two basic beliefs that I call the "minimum conception of a feminist ethics" must reject ethical vegetarianism. These two beliefs are: First, no ethics can permit arbitrariness in its prescriptions and theories. Second, any specifically feminist ethic must affirm the value of the female body. Whatever else a feminist ethics is or will be, it must reject requiring women to live as if physiologically identical to men and assigning arbitrary moral burdens to women or other persons based on factors that cannot be changed by human choice. My arguments show that all formulations of ethical vegetarianism, whether traditionalist or feminist, violate this "minimum conception."

The "vegan ideal" is not a *moral* ideal at all. Vegan diets may be adopted as a personal lifestyle, but a vegan moral ideal would idealize those of a particular age, sex, class, ethnicity, and culture; that is, adult (age 20–50), middle-class, mostly white males living in high-tech societies—the group with the most power in our world.

I believe that feminists should not moralize about food practice, even though it remains appropriate to condemn cruelty and to encourage moderation and semivegetarianism for that reason. This book shows you why I have come to believe that, at most, semivegetarian diets should be taught and that moral vegetarianism is inconsistent with feminism and is, in fact, at odds with the central assertions of feminism.

Chapter 2 reviews two of four major defenses of the claim that all or most humans ought to be vegetarians because animals have moral standing. I explain why traditional moral theory requires the equal consideration of nonhuman animals as well as ethical vegetarianism by summarizing the arguments of Tom Regan (1983) and Peter Singer (1975, 1990). Readers familiar with these arguments could easily skip these pages. Traditional virtue theory is also explained to distinguish it from rule-centered traditional ethics and to link it with some versions of contextual feminist ethics that will be discussed in the next chapter.

In chapter 3, I briefly review the recent arguments of some feminists and ecofeminists that feminism requires vegetarianism and probably veganism. Not all ecofeminists accept the logical connection of veganism and feminism, so I will attempt to give the most general tenets of ecofeminism first. Then I show how most of those who do link vegetarianism and feminism implicitly or explicitly depend upon the traditional moral arguments set out by Tom Regan,

Peter Singer, and others. Included in the discussion is the work of Carol Adams, Josephine Donovan, Marti Kheel, Deane Curtin, and others.

All four of the views in chapters 2 and 3 idealize the ethical vegetarian life as most virtuous, although Curtin's view is quite moderate. A "male physiological ideal" is assumed, however. That is, the adult male body is the moral norm. Chapter 4 presents the argument that all four defenses contain this hidden assumption. These four defenses also assume that living in cultures where adequate food and supplementation are available is not merely a health norm, but a moral norm as well. Regan, Singer, Adams, and Curtin rely on equality as sameness in the nutritional needs of males and females, children and the elderly. In making their moral arguments, these scholars must rely nutritional studies of adult males in industrialized countries. But they must ignore or dismiss studies and epidemiological evidence of the shortcomings of such diets for other age groups and for many women. The scientific norm is defined by the adult male body, which is less "vulnerable" to the adverse health consequences of vegetarian diets. If one argues for ethical vegetarianism based on the moral standing of animals, these moral arguments collapse because the claim is that *being less vulnerable is good,* simply because one is *stronger,* and *being vulnerable is bad* or, at least not as good, because one is *weaker.* A good moral argument should argue for justice, moral virtue, or caring rather than for simple physical force or power.

In later chapters, I will show why both traditional ethical defenses and feminist contextualist defenses fail. The supposed duty to be vegetarian relies on the false idea that the adult male body is, for practical nutritional purposes, the same as that of the adult female, the adolescent, the child, or the older person. It fails to recognize material differences among humans. If they wish to act rightly and yet accept this false belief, women, adolescents, children, the elderly, and others would be forced to suffer greater burdens than men, disadvantaging these groups with respect to health and economic power. That, in turn, perpetuates another false and unjust belief (or suspicion) that women and those who are less well off economically are *morally* weaker because they are *physically* weaker or live in circumstances without an industrialized food system. Here we see an example of how the powerful perpetuate their position through the structure of ethics itself.

In order to make the "male physiological norm" visible, a substantial portion of chapter 4 is devoted to discussion of the special nutritional needs of women, children, and the elderly. A cultural ideal of wealth and power is also embedded in ethical vegetarianism. To adumbrate this objectionable assumption, I also discuss various situations of nutritional vulnerability found in our own culture and in other cultures. The extended discussion of nutrition is intended to aid the concerned person who may be responsible for aging parents or young children. In my experience, those who are interested in the questions posed here want to understand the facts and are sincerely concerned to fulfill their moral responsibilities. Those who do not doubt the facts could easily skip the more scientific portions of chapter 4.

Those who may have questions and concerns about possible bias in the studies cited, mistakes in the reasoning, or conflicting nutritional information will find a discussion of these issues in the chapter 5.

In chapter 6, I discuss the ideas of equality and difference by review of some of recent feminist writings on the meaning of equality when gender differences require different rather than similar treatment. The assumed male norm becomes even more problematic in an ethic where species are unequal and one species cares for and uses the other. A feminist contextual ethics will be inadequate to ground an ethical vegetarian ideal because traditional patriarchal ideals and norms must be assumed in order to praise ethical vegetarianism. Thus, the ideal conflicts with the aims of ecofeminism and with the central claims of feminism in general.

In chapter 7, I elaborate my own view—that of *feminist aesthetic semivegetarianism*. I conclude that no justification or explanation whatever need be given by any *semivegetarian* regarding her eating habits. Nor should we praise or blame anyone for moderate meat and animal product consumption.

This book is a continuation of my attempt to make sense of my own beliefs about feminism, ethical vegetarianism, animal suffering, parenting, and the conflicting responsibilities that accepting these beliefs and responsibilities entails. I hope it will assist you in the same quest.

CHAPTER 2

ETHICAL VEGETARIANISM AND TRADITIONAL MORAL THEORY

THE RESURGENT INTEREST IN ETHICAL VEGETARIANISM

Ethical vegetarianism in various forms has been advocated by religious, moral, and health teachers since ancient times. In all major religions, those who have been able to live as vegetarians, or more ideally as vegans, have been regarded by the nonvegetarian faithful as living the highest life and being of the highest virtue (Spencer 1993). In Eurocentric culture, vegetarianism has a centuries-old association with spirituality and purity (Twigg 1979). Most contemporary Western writers who offer a systematic philosophical defense of ethical vegetarianism have used either utilitarian theory (for example, Singer 1975) or a deontological moral rights theory (for example, Regan 1983; Rollin 1981).[1]

A recent revival of virtue theory has occurred in traditional philosophy and some ecofeminists have articulated ethical positions whose structure resembles deontic and virtue approaches, reinterpreting these traditional arguments in a feminine or feminist voice. The rights arguments of Tom Regan and Bernard Rollin as well as the utilitarian arguments of Peter Singer have had the greatest social impact in the United States and parts of Europe in recent years. Ecofeminist arguments about obligations to animals are relatively new and have not yet reached a more general audience. Although most Americans remain omnivores, the controversy over "animal rights" is well-known to most adults (Groller 1990). National magazines such as *Newsweek* (Cowley *et al.* 1988,

Seligmann and Wright 1988, Begley 1990), the *New Republic* (Wright 1990), and the *Campus Voice* (Auchmutey 1986) have covered questions about animal rights and animal liberation. Network television periodically covers the maltreatment of animals in laboratories, feedlots, stockyards, and on farms.

Perhaps in response to this information, awareness of Americans concerning ethical arguments for vegetarianism has increased substantially over the past twenty years, although many people cite "health reasons" as the basis for their vegetarian preferences. Vegetarian alternatives do appear on most restaurant menus and are commonly offered now at academic meetings. According to Patricia K. Johnston (1994), "growing interest in vegetarian diets among the general population is reflected in recent surveys. One survey reported that as many as twenty percent of American adults are likely or very likely to look for a restaurant that serves vegetarian items when they decide to eat out. . . . Another survey found that 13.5 percent of all U.S. households claim to have at least one vegetarian member. This would mean there are some twelve million vegetarians nationwide. This represents an eightfold increase from 1979 to 1992" (vii). Peter Singer (1990) comments that even conservatives he meets are now apologetic about being omnivores, which is a testament to a growing thoughtfulness and concern about whether it is wrong to eat meat.

This chapter explains the arguments for ethical vegetarianism that are extended from traditional moral theory; that is, rights, utilitarianism, and virtue theories. Although numerous authors have defended versions of animal rights or welfare, I shall refer to the views of Singer (1975, 1986, 1990) and Regan (1983, 1991) almost exclusively, because their work is paradigmatically set within traditional moral theory and is best known to most readers. Some of the most common difficulties with these theories are also discussed. The next chapter explains the feminist and ecofeminist moral arguments. Chapters 4, 6 and 7 present detailed arguments about why neither traditional nor feminist moral arguments demand ethical vegetarianism.

DEFINING THE MORAL COMMUNITY

For the last two hundred years philosophers have approached ethics with certain assumptions: reason gives truth, whereas emotion does not; rules are required for rational justification of moral choices; and moral thinking itself must be hierarchically structured. The ideal human being has been held up as primarily differentiated and "free" (as opposed to related or dependent), individualistic, albeit self-interested and self-seeking, atavistic, power-oriented, and male. This view of human nature reflects the self-concept of the ideal man of the dominant class. In addition, philosophers debate whether utilitarianism, rights, or virtue theory is the correct *method* to employ in ethical decision making. Since that time philosophers and society at large have engaged in a long discussion of who should be accorded moral equality. Recent philosophical discussion in animal rights and animal welfare treats questions of method and of moral standing as conceptually distinct (Regan 1983; Singer 1975, 1986, 1990); that is, the question of which moral theory is the correct one is separate from that of "who counts?" as an equal in the moral community.

Feminists have argued that reliance on these traditional Enlightenment categories, hierarchies, and dichotomies is typical of thought systems articulated almost exclusively by the dominant, mostly white male class. But the opposition of reason to emotion denies the epistemic quality of emotion and its ethical content. Moreover, the current conception of human nature does not encompass the perspectives of the subordinate or the ruled. Nevertheless, those who advocate all or part of the moral tradition may well be feminists of any gender who are struggling with ways to understand and revise ethical thought and decision making. Perhaps with the advance of a "strong objectivity" (Harding 1991), a more inclusive ethics can be expected to supersede older, narrower views.

WHO COUNTS?

Before deciding which moral approach to use, we must *first* settle questions about whom our decision applies to, their relationship with us, and the basis for our considering them or not. Traditional philosophers phrase this as a concern about who counts in the moral community. Typically, definitional approaches are used to try to decide who belongs and who doesn't. The philosopher tries to discover some property common to all members of the known class (that is, those we are sure should be members). Then she uses it as a standard against which to decide whether some or all of those in question also share that characteristic and so should be included, too.[2] For many centuries thinkers in ethics have been debating who belongs in the class of *equals*. The ancient aristocracies fell in the social, political, and religious movements to break down class barriers. Thus, Mary Wollstonecraft (1792) argued that women should have equal rights on the grounds that women are capable of the same thought and reason as men. Abolitionists argued against slavery. In *The Expanding Circle* (1981), Peter Singer argues that recent history shows that the scope of equality is increasing. In ancient times, only male citizens were regarded as peers, but with the overthrow of monarchies in Europe, even the lowliest common white male was given a voice and considered the equal of the wealthy and strong. Later, other races were included, and women were emancipated. Now the circle is expanding to nonhuman animals and to nature itself.

Both Peter Singer (1975) and Tom Regan (1983) attempt to show that "all animals are equal" and that humans have moral duties or obligations to at least some nonhuman animals. Such animals are dubbed "members of the moral community." A "moral community" differs from other communities because, unlike a village or a town, it has no geographical location. It resembles a religious community in that the members (Hindus, Christians, Muslims, Jews and so forth) could be anywhere in the world. What binds a religious community together is common beliefs and desires rather than any physical characteristic as such. And there is a notion of inclusion and exclusion: some are members, some are not. The *moral* community is larger, though, and includes at least all members of religious communities as well as all of the irreligious. Even atheists and criminals belong (Feinberg 1973; Vlastos 1962). Only a single general belief holds this community together—that there are some things that may not be done to a member without very good reasons; concomitant with and foundational to that belief is the affirmation of life and the condemnation of needless suffering.

Singer and Regan employ a similar philosophical method for rational determination of whether animals have the *essential* characteristics of members. First, each looks as the "paradigm class," noting the common observable features of those who already have rights or who are counted in a utilitarian calculus. Common features of the class that is proposed for admission are then compared with similar features of the paradigm class, first, for their presence or absence, and second, for their relevance to morality. If essential, relevant features are present and not absent, then the beings in the paradigm class and those in the proposed class are similar "where it matters" for morality. Singer, Regan, and virtually every other author arguing for inclusion of nonhuman animals as equals recite the various *material* similarities and differences among human and nonhuman animals, noting that most historically cited differences do not now stand up to philosophical scrutiny. Differences have often served as grounds for exclusion from the class of *moral* equals and as justification for unequal and unfair treatment. Nonhuman animals have been held *un*equal for a variety of reasons, among them: (1) Only humans are rational, and rationality is essential to membership; (2) only humans are moral, and humans have duties only to other beings with moral responsibilities; (3) only humans have souls, and we have duties only to those with souls; in the same vein (4) only humans have language; (5) only humans think; (6) only humans are self-aware; (7) only humans value their own lives; (8) only humans are "ends-in-themselves" (Kant

1785); (9) only humans feel pain (Descartes as well as a myriad of behavioral psychologists and other animal researchers; see Rollin 1989).

The idea of species equality is foundational to all arguments for the rights, welfare, and liberation of animals. Singer argues that failure to regard animals as full members of the moral community is "speciesism" and is wrong in the same way that racism and sexism are wrong (1975, 7). Both utilitarians and rights advocates accept similar notions of species equality—that the interests of all animals in avoiding death and suffering are of equal importance. The qualities considered most relevant for defining these interests are discussed further in the sections on "Utilitarianism" and "Deontological Ethics and Rights" below.

RULES AND JUSTICE

Having determined which features are most important for membership, the next step is to consider what justice demands when the relevant features of particular individuals are considered. Religious and secular teachers alike have traditionally referred to rules as the central guide to justice in both morality and law. The Ten Commandments, the Principle of Utility, and the Categorical Imperative are among the best-known examples of moral rules. The importance of legal rules traces to the most ancient times where the moral law became public in the Code of Hammurabi, Hebrew law, and later Roman law. Morality and legality are not co-extensive, but a discussion of their differences would take us too far afield. Here, I point to the antiquity of rules because their durability in ethical thinking makes them more stubbornly ingrained and more difficult to see beyond.

Within deontological ethics at least, a fundamental rule of justice is that "like cases should be treated alike." So, for example, women and men should receive the same basic consideration when applying for jobs, education, and other opportunities. Newborns should not be summarily killed because their existence is inconvenient for parents or society, and the retarded should not be experimented upon, made to suffer, or used for purposes that do not primarily benefit them as individuals. The rule or principle of equality demands such equal consideration based on factors other than gender, age, race, class, and so forth. Differing treatment based on individual differences in experience, education, and capacities may be considered appropriate, but discrimination on the basis of *simple* difference is objectionable because gender, age, race, and so forth are regarded as irrelevant to other moral concerns. Moral theorists usually argue that, in an ideal society, these characteristics ought to be irrelevant to the realization of a particular person's highest good. I interpret this to mean at minimum that equality affirms the *quality* of a life in its individuality. "Quality" is defined as "that which makes something what it is" and "the degree of excellence of a thing" (Webster's 1971); thus, as applied to beings for whom realization of their own good is possible, equality should be thought of as weighting that quality the same among them. That is, the good of such beings is of similar importance to each being itself, and moral respect requires that each of us care about such a good.

Such an understanding of equality and a morality based upon it departs in important ways from usages that refer to "equal rights" or "equal consideration under the law." Such usages emphasize the similar application of laws and rules to faceless persons who present themselves as enmeshed in situations chronic to the human condition. The laws themselves are supposed to operate similarly, or equally, in such cases. Thus, laws are generated to deal with recurrent conditions that are described in general terms and are often regarded as "universal" in that similar problems occur in cultures separated by time and geography. A law is applied equally and justice is said to be served, say, if all bank robbers performing holdups in virtually the same circumstances receive the same due process and criminal punishment. The rule operates the same for all.

In the usage I wish to presuppose, beings themselves are supposed to be equals in that their lives and their own good are seen as intrinsically worthwhile. As I will explain in chapter 6, the presence of a plurality of values and norms threatens to make the notion of equality unworkable.

THE RULE-BASED EGALITARIAN MORAL TRADITION

THE "COMMON SENSE" VIEW

Cruelty to animals is recognized as wrongful in all cultures, although what counts as cruelty may vary. The Bible contains many admonitions against cruelty to animals.[3] Introducing a volume discussing the religious perspectives of Judaism, Christianity, Islam, Hinduism, Buddhism, Jainism, and Confucianism, John Bowker (1986) summarizes what all of the religions agree about concerning the use of animals:

> First, all religions agree that their traditions do not have a concept of animal *rights* but that animals do have valid claims upon us. Second, they agree that to ignore those claims, or to regard them as trivial . . . , is to do long-term damage to the stature of being human. . . . Third, they agree that the validity of the claim of animals upon us is reinforced—perhaps even grounded—in the sense of the unity of life. . . . Fourth, they agree that death is not the

greatest evil one can imagine . . . or conversely, that there are or may be more important things in life than living. Fifth, they agree that the various uses of animals must be differentiated: *some* uses *may* be justified, whereas others cannot be. Therefore, sixth, they agree that the cultivation of pity, compassion, identification, and sympathy for animals is not, *ipso facto*, an expression of the pathetic fallacy but a necessary part of growing up (11–12).

In the Western nations, Christianity, its thinkers, and its theologians have had the greatest influence on human attitudes toward animals, especially domestic species. Saint Augustine, Saint Thomas Aquinas, and Immanuel Kant all commented on the nature of our obligations to animals. Until the nineteenth century the common sense view of animals' place in the moral community was one that prohibited cruelty. Animals were regarded as "naturally under slavery" and placed on the earth by God for use by humans. As Bernard Rollin (1989) has argued, ordinary people have always known that animals feel pain and even a common sense view of morality prohibits inflicting unnecessary pain. Augustine in the fifth century A.D. and Aquinas in the thirteenth century wrestled with the problem of killing "dumb beasts," justifying their use by appeal to the claim that an animal's nature makes it something to be used by humans. As I use it here, the "anti–cruelty view," whether linked to religion or not, refers to the idea that animals have a subordinate place to humans in moral decision making. Cruelty is wrong, and cruelty consists in inflicting needless pain and suffering to any being capable of feeling it. Not all suffering is cruel, however, because various justifications are accepted for causing another being pain. Although a full discussion of the justifications for inflicting pain is not possible here, examples include inflicting a short term pain to prevent or alleviate long–term suffering, punishing those guilty of transgressions of morality, voluntarily accepting pain to achieve a valued goal, and so forth. Therefore, in the anti–cruelty view, some values are more important than pain and suffering and are worthwhile achieving in spite of or even because of suffering. Thus, the simple ability to suffer or feel pain would not serve as an adequate defining criterion for *equal* membership in the moral community, although pain is regarded as morally relevant. The anti–cruelty view refers to the idea that the good of nonhuman animals is morally important, but less important than the full realization of the good of human beings. Animals will not be the equal of humans.

Peter Singer, Bernard Rollin, Tom Regan, Steven Sapontzis (1987), Andrew Linzey (1987) and the many other modern thinkers who write in defense of nonhuman animals do not take the anti–cruelty view and argue against it vigorously.

UTILITARIANISM

In *Animal Liberation* Peter Singer (1975) exposed the cruelty of scientific experimentation on animals and the callous attitudes of some researchers of the time. In the first part of the book, Singer argues that "all animals are equal," and the basis for their equality is the capacity to feel pain. In matters where lives are at stake, Singer (1975) adds "self-awareness, intelligence, [and] the capacity for meaningful relations with others" as criteria for decision making (21); thus, a normal adult pig should not be killed, in Singer's view, to save the life of a severely retarded child, but may be killed to save the life of a normal human. All other differences between human and nonhuman animals are morally irrelevant. Then, using the methodology of classical utilitarian theory, he argues for the injustice of and abolition of hunting, trapping, experimentation with animals, animal farming, and for universal vegetarianism based on animal rights.[4]

Singer (1975) revives Jeremy Bentham's (1789) concern for animal pain and with it the question of which criteria we should use to decide who counts as an equal. For a consistent utilitarian, pleasure and pain, as abstract things which can be experienced by any sentient being, are all that matter for morality. Bentham and, subsequently, Singer hold that capacities to experience pleasure and pain determine who belongs to the moral community, and clearly a large number of animal species can experience pain and so must be counted.[5]

Utilitarian methodology appears relatively simple. Once a utilitarian knows generally who is to be counted in the decision making process, she must consider her alternatives and the sensitive beings who will be affected by each of her possible choices. Then, for each alternative she is to sum up the pleasure and the pain that would result for each being involved, including herself. No one is to be given special consideration. Then, she is to compare all the alternatives and choose the one that promotes the "greatest good for the greatest number." Utilitarianism is future-oriented; only the consequences of actions count rather than intentions. Although decisionmakers cannot be expected to make an exact quantification of pleasure and pain, utilitarians claim that we do have a "rough and ready" idea of the relative pleasure and pain we cause others with our choices. Bentham equated "interests" with whatever is pleasurable or painful for an individual. A right action is the sum of the interests of the individuals in the community.

DEONTOLOGICAL ETHICS AND RIGHTS

Bernard Rollin (1981) and Tom Regan (1983) argue that animals have all the essential characteristics necessary for membership in the moral community and that they therefore have certain rights not to suffer harm or death.[6] Their commitment to rights rather than utilitarianism follows the deontological tradition of many religions. A rule-based deontic ethics sets forth certain imperatives, principles, or commandments that a person is expected to follow regardless of whether it seems to maximize happiness or the general good at the time. Rights are often contrasted to utility as affording better protection for individuals in the pursuit of unpopular ideas: a majority committed to respecting rights may be unhappy about the religious beliefs of a minority group, but should still refrain from persecuting them for their beliefs.[7]

Early rights advocates did not think nonhuman animals could have rights. In his *Lectures on Ethics*, Immanuel Kant (1780) specifically argued against the inclusion of animals in the moral community and held that only rational agents can be of concern to us. Humans have a dignity and intrinsic moral worth *because* they are rational and can make moral choices. But, Kant argued, "so far as animals are concerned, we have no direct duties. Animals are not self-conscious and are there merely as means to an end. That end is man" (1780, 239). Thus, nonhuman animals are not worthy of respect for their own sake. They have neither dignity nor intrinsic worth, and Kant viewed them as only instruments with a price. We do have "indirect duties" to them, however, given that we have duties to humans. People who are cruel to animals, Kant thought, might also be cruel to humans; thus, for the sake of the humans, we should be kind to animals. This rationalization is sometimes found in defenses of the anti–cruelty view.

In *The Case for Animal Rights*, Regan (1983) shows why Kant's criterion of rational agency fails as a necessary ground for having rights: many "marginal case" humans (infants, retarded persons, the senile) lack rational agency, and yet we would surely agree that they have rights (1983, 151–56; 260–62). It is enough to be a "subject-of-a-life." Being a "subject" means having a range of intelligence and sensitivity (to pain, suffering, and other psychological experiences) such that it matters to the being itself what is done to it. Humans and animals alike suffer pain and have interests in not being harmed, killed, or having their important preferences frustrated (also see Rollin 1989). Regan finds that being a mammal at least one year of age is generally sufficient to guarantee subjectivity. Subjects have a good of their own and thus have what Regan terms "inherent value." Inherent value is contrasted with the "instrumental value" that tools and other mere objects have. So, we should regard other people and animals who are "subjects-of-a life" not merely as tools for our use but as good-in-themselves (1983, 243–48).

In essence, Regan retains Kant's distinction about some beings having merely a price whereas others have dignity, but Regan argues that animals have dignity, too. Thus, they have certain rights protecting their own good. In the categorical nature of the rights he claims for animals, Regan is thoroughly Kantian and dualistic in his metaphysics.

Singer and Regan *agree* that animals share with us a degree of intelligence and sensitivity and that they therefore have "welfare interests."[8] For Regan, "welfare-interests" are those things that are good for an individual regardless of whether the being knows or desires these things—for instance, life, health, security. Regan distinguishes these from "preference-interests," which the being may desire but may or may not contribute to or be necessary for well-being (1983, 87–88). Their having welfare-interests and capacities makes animals as well as humans members of the moral community. For Regan, this means the members have rights. In traditional moral theory, some rights—such as rights not to be killed and rights not to be harmed—are very stringently protected, although they are almost never absolute or exceptionless.[9] They are held equally by all members.[10] We might suppose that some beings are superior to others, have more rights, or different rights, but as Regan (1983) points out, what morally relevant difference can be used to make this distinction? Higher intelligence is often cited; but, even if animals are less intelligent than humans, this merely gives humans more power, not more worth. Singer (1975) ties interests to satisfaction of real needs and desires of the organism, and his view of interests parallels Regan's. The primary differences between them arise in the way one is to decide what to do—sum utility interests in alternative moral scenarios or protect interests with adherence to deontological rules known as rights.

Most rights advocates, including Rollin and Regan, regard interests in life, security, and freedom from harm as most important and generating the most stringent of rights. Justifications for waiver or override of such rights are limited: for example, concerning the right not to be killed, persons guilty of murder may be punished or even executed. Killing in self-defense usually is permitted, but the burden of proof falls heavily on the defender. These limitations protect the innocent against punishment for crimes and offenses which she or he did not commit and from homicides for frivolous reasons. Waiver and override requirements are especially stringent when the other has no bad intent—something that domestic food animals do not have. Self-defense also implies some clear danger that justifies the defender's action. Animal rights are meant to protect nonhuman animals from arbitrary harm and killing: if animals have rights, it is wrong to confine them and exploit them for our pleasure, convenience, or economic good.

WHY VEGETARIANISM IS MORALLY REQUIRED

Singer's (1975) utilitarian method would allow some animals and/or humans to be killed for the greater good, but he argues for ethical vegetarianism on the grounds that we have no real need (and so, no welfare-interest) for meat or animal products. Our predilections for them are merely matters of taste. These latter interests are of lesser value and cannot outweigh an animal's welfare interest in life and freedom from the confinement practices used to produce their products. Regan (1983) argues that all or almost all moral people must become vegetarians because animals have rights not to be killed and used for food. Because animals have such rights, food animal production, hunting, trapping, and the use of animals in research must be abolished, he claims. Regan has clearly influenced many people to adopt ethical veganism, and he follows a vegan diet himself. His rights arguments do not require such strict adherence, however. He claims that only mammals one year of age or older can be clearly defined as subjects-of-a-life. Presumably, eating veal, chicken and other birds, fish, reptiles, and "lower" animals (or even human infants) would be permissible, but Regan argues that such animals should not be consumed either (1983, 349, 367). He asserts that we ought to grant these animals the benefit of the doubt about subjectivity, although he says little about the ground for such doubts. In addition, he argues that we should not eat animal products because they are inhumanely produced. On the question of whether human infants count, Regan notes that the "subject-of-a-life" criterion is merely a sufficient condition for membership in the class of rights-holders. Other sufficient conditions might be found; thus, it does not follow that infants must lack rights. He has also drawn the specific line at "mammals one year of age or older" for the sake of proceeding with his argument. Below that line he claims that we are not very sure about the being's subjectivity, but this uncertainty means that some who fall below the line, such as infants, could also be subjects. Finally, he argues that we have a duty to maintain a moral climate in which rights are taken seriously, and it would be important to give infants "the benefit of the doubt, viewing them *as if* they are subjects-of-a-life, *as if* they have basic rights, even while conceding that, in viewing them in these ways, we may be giving them more than is their due" (Regan, 319–20). This latter point—that infants merely receive "the benefit of the doubt"—exposes the heart of the difference between traditional moral theories and feminine or feminist theories of care, where the mother-child relationship is the moral paradigm. I personally cannot conceive of doubting the moral standing of my child.

Regan seems to think that his position admits very few exceptions. His argument relies on an empirical nutritional claim that almost all humans can live well on vegan diets. Exceptions to the rule of moral vegetarianism are granted to those who would be harmed by such diets, but Regan apparently believes that only a relatively small number of people would count as such "exceptional cases," especially in industrialized countries where food and supplements are widely available.

Regan's arguments also depend on universality, equality under the moral law, and the "vegan ideal." The rights are universal—their proscriptions and protections apply to everyone. Like cases should be treated alike, and rights should protect animals and humans equally. In a more perfect society, all virtuous persons would live in accordance with a "vegan ideal" lifestyle. Similarly, Singer also follows a vegan diet and argues that the vegan ideal is most virtuous and is required by utilitarianism. Therefore, both argue that food animal farming, experimentation with animals, hunting, trapping, and all other exploitive uses of animals must cease (Regan) or be drastically curtailed (Singer). Regan and Singer agree that equality, impartiality, and universality require ethical vegetarianism.

TRADITIONAL PROBLEMS WITH THE TRADITIONAL MORAL THEORIES

INTERPRETING MORAL RESPECT

Accounting for the dignity and worth of members of the moral community has presented difficulties for modern utilitarians. Peter Singer (1975) acknowledges the value of a virtue that has been called "moral respect" and agrees that it is wrong to use animals simply as tools. As a moral theory, utilitarianism offers little "logical space" for including this kind of virtue, though. Methodological considerations of summing the interests of individuals to calculate the good should prevent the utilitarian from concern for the interests of particular beings unless such concern would ultimately serve the overall good. Individuals are, at best, of derivative importance (Smart and Williams 1973). In his (1979) Singer wrestles with the "replaceability argument"—a problem inherent to utilitarianism in general: if happiness, pleasure, satisfaction, suffering, and pain are the only measures of good and evil, it would not appear to be wrong to painlessly kill an infant, an adult, or an animal as long as we replace the being with another infant or animal who is equally happy.[11] Yet, this is patently wrong. Immanuel Kant and Tom Regan can appeal to their view of persons to explain why: particular persons (including mammals one year old for Regan) are "above all price," they are irreplaceable, and their relative happiness or unhappiness does not diminish their intrinsic worth or their dignity. Singer (1986) admits that he can find no satisfactory answer to this problem within utilitarian theory. Singer's acknowledgment that sensitive beings should not to be used as mere tools nor be summarily replaced by equally happy beings shows that he is indebted to Kant as well as to Bentham. The interests of humans and animals are to be conceived of in noninstrumental ways, making Singer's conception of interests quite similar, if not identical, with that of Regan and other rights thinkers.

SOME CONCERNS ABOUT INTERESTS

The concept of interests is central in these traditional moral theories. As mentioned above, Bentham equated "interests" with whatever is pleasurable or painful for an individual. A right action is the sum of the interests of the individuals in the community. Bentham's notion of interests was not well-developed. R. M. Hare (1981) and others in the past several decades have substituted the raw notions of pleasure and pain and satisfaction of desires with a richer concept of "interests" than Bentham imagined, and we may safely assume that Singer and Regan are well-versed in this literature.

Traditionalists recognize a general difficulty with saying a person has an interest in whatever she finds pleasurable: moralists seem to be committed to permitting satisfaction of some rather base desires. Should we maximize a masochist's opportunities for his pleasures and the opportunities of a sadistic majority to persecute an unfortunate minority? No. Hare (1981) argues that only people's "perfectly prudent preferences" should be maximized—those that we would have if we were fully informed about what is really in the interests of ourselves and others, where an interest is something that is truly good for a person. John Harsanyi (1982) concurs: "In deciding what is good and what is bad for an individual, the ultimate criterion can only be his wants and his own preferences" (55). But Harsanyi allows that "his own preferences [may be] at some deeper level . . . inconsistent with what he is now trying to achieve" so that we simply have to "distinguish between a person's manifest preferences and his true preferences" and these are the ones "he *would* have if he had all the relevant information, always reasoned with the greatest possible care, and were in a state of mind most conducive to rational choice" (55).

Although Harsanyi's (1982) solution seems reasonable at first, Amartya Sen and Bernard Williams (1982) show that it assumes what it attempts to prove. Harsanyi (1982) and Hare (1981) beg the question because they simply rule out ahead of time all "antisocial preferences, such as sadism, envy, resentment, and malice [as] . . . irrational" (56) without explaining why such preferences should

be thought so. By analogy, Singer makes a similar mistake. He rules out preferences for meat and animal products as irrational by definition and therefore not
in the true interest of human beings.

Similarly, "perfectly prudent preferences" bear a striking resemblance to what
Regan (1983), Feinberg (1984), VanDeVeer (1979), and others have referred to
as "welfare-interests"—they are more than whatever interests the being has but
instead consist in what a being would want if she or he had perfect knowledge
of her own good. Roughly speaking, then, an interest is something that is truly
good for a being whether the being knows it or not. This brings us back to
square one—what is truly good for humans or for nonhumans, for that matter?
It was supposed to be our preferences, but it turns out that only some of these
preferences really count, and on reflection only these constitute our "interests."

A further problem concerns evaluating the interests of individuals and
including them in the utilitarian calculus: Suppose we simply try to maximize
the preferences of the moral community. We do not summarily rule out preferences for meat and instead give those desires some consideration. We also give
animal suffering a negative value. When we try to sum up alternative utilities,
we will have to assume that the preferences of everyone affected will take on relatively the same shape or form; that is, that preferences will not be so conflicting as to defeat any possible decision making. J. A. Mirrlees (1982) points out
that this assumption is often false, particularly in our own society. That being
so, "in extreme cases, it may be that there are no grounds for moral choice at
all" (84). Notwithstanding these difficulties, traditional morality requires that
we act in the true (or objective) interests of others, not merely what we think
they might want at the time. To do that, we must have some idea of what
objective interests are, that is, of what is generally good for humans and animals
(and arguably other entities as well).

HUMAN NATURE, ESSENTIALISM, AND EQUALITY

To have an objective interest presupposes having a common human or species
nature.[12] Human nature has usually been thought of as *teleological*. Humans are
said to have a particular goal, aim, or *raison d'être*. The better ways of living are
to be sought and the worse avoided. Moral teachers prescribe rules, attitudes,
and practices to be adopted that allow the full flourishing of one's best self,
while warning students away from corrupting evils. Often, a quality unique to
humans, separating them from other species, was designated as the special
interest to be developed. Thus, reason or rationality is to be cultivated according to Plato and Aristotle. Aristotle argued that reason and speech are the

essence of human nature because these qualities are particular to humans and set them apart from animals. Christian thinkers identified the soul (enclosed in a weak and selfish body) as the essence of humanity, and the virtues of faith, hope, love, and obedience are extolled as the way to the highest life.

In the pre-Darwinian Christian world, distinctive differences isolated one species from another as God's "special creations." Positing equality based on species identity (all and only humans are equal) seemed to present little difficulty. After Darwin, species do not present themselves as materially discrete entities. All living things have DNA, and all the heretofore uniquely human qualities such as sentience, emotions, communication, and problem-solving appear in many non-human animals as well. The species are related to one another on a genetic tree, and the differences among us are not in kind, but only in degree. Attempts to draw a line dividing beings who count from those who do not at the human species barrier seem arbitrary because *moral equality* has heretofore been argued for on the basis of *material equality*. Equal justice means that similar forms shall receive similar treatment; like cases shall be treated alike.

To argue for species equality, Singer and Regan presuppose a common animal nature, some essence of what it is to be a living, feeling being. This likeness among humans and nonhumans must provide an adequate basis for morality. At the same time, the logic of traditional moral theory commits them to a notion of the good that is virtually universal for humans and for animals. The good of a being may vary from species to species and with circumstances, but a thoughtful moral traditionalist must recognize some conception of "welfare" that would be meaningless apart from such interspecies understanding. Further, the interests connected to that common animal nature must be equally considered. That is, the pain and suffering of animals, their interests, the particular good of these beings is to be valued equally with that of human beings. And these shared interests are to take precedence over the *differences* in interests that humans and nonhumans may have. I shall return to a discussion of similarity and difference in chapter 6.

SOME CONCERNS ABOUT PRACTICE

Some critics charge that utilitarianism is epistemically impoverished by its reliance on calculation—if hanging an innocent person would prevent riots and several deaths, should the authorities proceed? Deontology is similarly afflicted by the lack of criteria to decide a case when two equally important moral rules compete—should one keep a promise to return a weapon if in the meantime the person has gone mad and threatens others? Feminists often object that too much moral attention is focused on abstract conceptions of rights, interests, and obligations. In the attempt to be unbiased, too many of the particularities of the real life context are lost. Other important aspects of morality, such as relationship, love, and personal goodness languish and seem forgotten. While the emphasis on sensitivity and pain in utilitarianism may seem to encourage people to place themselves in the shoes of others, contemporary traditionalist thinkers argue that caring, personal relationships, and personal virtue have no privileged role in utilitarian theory (Slote 1985, 1992; Kultgen 1998a,b). Classically, Bentham roundly condemned setting up laws and moral rules based in mere personal feelings of "sympathy and antipathy"— that is, of love and hate, approval and disapproval. Bentham was intent on condemning the actions of tyrants and all old systems of morality as being based on arbitrary personal feelings. Such laws served the classes in power and not human beings in general. He argued that all other moral systems "consist all of them in so many contrivances for avoiding the obligation of appealing to any external standard, and for prevailing upon the reader to accept of the author's sentiment or opinion as a reason for itself" (1789, 50). While Bentham is surely right in condemning a morality constructed on arbitrary and self-serving privilege and power, he is surely wrong in supposing that the emotions should be excised from moral epistemology.

Why don't these theories work well in contexts or ordinary situations? The reasons are many, but Rosemarie Tong (1993) tells the story of her own experience with unmodified traditional moral theory. She went into graduate school to study traditional ethical theory quite hopeful of being able to conceive of a moral theory that was "equally attentive to the consequences of and motives for actions; it would be no more concerned about group happiness than about individual rights; and it would bring everyone somehow closer together" (23). What discouraged her was not so much an inability to resolve these two competing moral theories, but their lack of application to the real life cases that occur in our lives every day.[13] Each of these theories has the unnerving capacity to be short-circuited. For example, utilitarianism depends on the calculation of the sum of pleasure and pain units for various courses of action and this procedure can have some unsettling outcomes. As Bernard Williams has said, a really moral person regards some situations as unthinkable. "For him, there are certain situations so monstrous that the idea that the processes of moral rationality could yield an answer in them is insane: they are situations which so transcend in enormity the human business of moral deliberation that from a moral point of view it cannot matter any more what happens . . . unless the environment reveals minimum sanity, it is insanity to carry the decorum of sanity into it.

Consequentialist rationality, however, and in particular utilitarian rationality, has no such limitations: making the best of a bad job is one of its maxims, and it will have something to say even on the difference between massacring seven million, and massacring seven million and one" (Smart and Williams 1973, 92). Similarly, Michael Slote (1985) has discussed the problem that utilitarians do not seem to have justification for caring more about one's own projects and one's own family than for others'. Schneewind (1990) notes that "Benthamite utilitarianism has, of course, no room for virtues in the traditional sense. It provides a rational decision procedure for every case, so that there is no room for the imprecisions of the imperfect duties, still less for the insight of the virtuous agent, or for any attribution of value to certain kinds of character other than an instrumental value in reliably producing good results" (57).

While many feminists argue that morality should have its basis in caring and relationship, deontologists generally reject relationship, love, or caring as bases for decision making: "Kant can make no room for love. Love as inclination or feeling or tender sympathy is dismissed in one sentence. It cannot be commanded. It must be replaced by 'beneficence from duty' . . ." (Schneewind 1990, 58). However, further general criticisms of rights and utilitarianism are many and would take us too far afield here. Those who wish to review them should see Smart and Williams (1973); Rachels (1986); and for the feminist concerns, Tong (1993). I will return to some specific concerns as they affect arguments for ethical vegetarianism in the following chapters.

TRADITIONAL VIRTUE ETHICS

The third approach to ethics is both older and newer than the theoretical approaches discussed above—older because virtually everyone writing in traditional virtue ethics acknowledges a debt to the ancient Greeks and to Aristotle, in particular. In fact, "the prospect of recovering an Aristotelian ethics of virtue, or something very like it, is a common thread of contemporary virtue ethics" (Hittinger 1989, 452). And virtue ethics is newer in that the project of "recovery" is relatively recent and has been complicated by the necessity of reconciling the "primacy of the virtuous" with other concerns better expressed by the deontological or utilitarian traditions (Garcia 1990).[14] That is, in a virtue ethics, character traits must be considered the foundation of ethics rather than rules or commandments. The revival is new enough that the concepts of virtue and vice are often unfamiliar to undergraduates and their parents alike. In what follows, I will explain virtue ethics by contrasting it to the ethics of duty. Then I will explain some aspects of modern virtue ethics that differ from Aristotelian virtue ethics.

Third, I will present some criticism or "doubts" about this moral framework. Finally, I explain how nineteenth and twentieth century vegetarianism relates to virtue, as a prelude to chapter 3, which covers feminism and vegetarianism.

Contrast to Ethics of Duty

What is the difference between virtue ethics and the approaches discussed earlier? And would this approach be more fruitful for incorporation of moral vegetarianism into an ethical life? The ethics of duty—rights, utilitarianism, and theocentric or deontic ethics—usually does not exclude the virtues.[15] In an ethics of duty, acts and decisions are good or evil or right or wrong, and these are judged to be so according to whether one follows a valid moral rule such as the Principle of Utility or a Kantian imperative or a justified right. A utilitarian would claim that acts bringing pleasure or the satisfaction of desire or preferences are good, and virtuous people continuously practice right actions which follow from the Principle of Utility. Similarly, rights thinkers and other neo-Kantians would claim that consistent and continuous adherence to the imperatives of duty expressed by the valid rules will be necessary and sufficient to inform the character of any person.[16] Such repetitions of rule-following will make her a good person, or at least a better person than she would be were she to set out simply to emulate others she admires without justificatory (rule-driven) understanding about why she will be a better person.

But virtue ethics arises from a wholly different outlook and history. In Western society we usually think of ethics as having to do with right and wrong and with duties, obligations, and responsibilities. But ancient thinkers did not write about duty. Plato, Aristotle, Epicurus, and the Stoics wrote about human excellence, pleasure, happiness, friendship, and the good life. Their approach is referred to as "virtue ethics." A virtuous person, according to Aristotle, aspires to realize his humanity, to perfect himself in accordance with his function or purpose as a human. For Aristotle, there were ideal ways to be human and an *essential* human nature—something that human beings are meant to be and become. He believed that man's essence is his rationality and that those who develop their rational powers to the highest degree fulfill their unique function *as humans*.[17] Such a person leads the highest life and is most likely to be happy and to feel the highest kind of human pleasure. This state of fulfillment is known as *eudaemonia*, a Greek word that cannot be translated by any single English word (see Aristotle 1984).

For the Greeks, the question for ethics was not "what is right and wrong?" but "how shall we live?" Aristotle accepted the idea that each kind of thing has an essential nature that is functional or teleological. A good thing of its kind, such as a winning race horse, is good because it performs its function well—in the case of the horse, it runs well. Likewise, a good sculptor sculpts well, and a good physician is able to heal his patients (Aristotle 1984). Each thing naturally strives to perfect itself in that function. Likewise, Aristotle argued that good, virtuous people are examples of such well-functioning, or as modern Aristotelians say, of human "flourishing." In the *Nichomachean Ethics*, Aristotle explores the nature of human excellence or virtue. He believed that human beings exist *for* some end, and human beings should use their capacity for reason to understand what that purpose is. In Book X of the *Nichomachean Ethics*, he argues that the highest life involves thinking about thinking, contemplation, or the philosophical life. Aristotle did not believe that his concept of human flourishing and human nature were social constructions or ideas that arose out of the presuppositions of the society into which he was born (Aristotle 1984).

To understand the difference between virtue ethics and duty ethics, think of what a person *is* rather than what she *does*. Rule-based duty ethics makes judgments of right acts primary and virtues derivative, whereas virtue ethics regards the moral character of persons as fundamental (Taylor 1991; Trianosky 1990; Garcia 1990; Montague 1992; Slote 1992; Kultgen 1998a,b). As Gregory Trianosky (1990) explains, "a pure ethics of virtue . . . claims that at least some judgments about virtue can be validated independently of any appeal to judgments about the rightness of actions . . . [and] . . . it is this antecedent goodness of traits which ultimately makes any right act right" (336). So, we are to look first at the person and her character to decide about the morality of her actions. We would look for honesty, courage, loyalty, and other virtues that would make her a good person. Presumably, a perfectly good person would be incapable of voluntarily committing a bad action. Of course, the ancient Greeks did not suppose any human could be perfectly good, but only that humans strive for it.

Particular dispositions to act in certain ways in certain situations are what Aristotle called virtues and vices. A truly virtuous person must know that what he does is right, he must choose it freely, and the action must come from a good character. On the last point, one cannot be called courageous for having done only one courageous act. Good character is informed by habitual practice of many acts of courage, large and small. In his explication of the Doctrine of the Mean, Aristotle names two kinds of virtues: intellectual virtues and moral virtues. Every good person must be have both of these kinds of virtue. The former are learned through a teacher and involve using one's reason to bring the passions and appetites into the range of the Mean of virtue. The moral virtues are such character traits as courage, piety, loyalty, fortitude, truthfulness and others. These are acquired by acts of practicing them until finally these actions become habitual. Only with practice will these virtues become so ingrained that finally the good person can simply act with virtue and will not necessarily need to ponder what to do in moments of crisis. Aristotle argued that the virtuous person (one possessing practical wisdom) would be happy (unless some catastrophe beyond his control should occur that plunged him into poverty, grief, or illness, for instance).

Modern Aristotelians or virtue ethicists usually want to keep some of Aristotle's ideas and abandon others. Today, most feminists and many traditionalists would wish to reject at least two of Aristotle's central ideas: (1) that human beings are innately unequal, and (2) that there is some essential and fixed human nature. Correlative to the latter is the rejection of the idea that women and men are essentially different and therefore should have different social roles and express different character traits.

Aristotle lived in an aristocratic society. He could not have conceived of the equal worth of all humans. Richard Taylor (1991) explains that "the concept of virtue . . . had originally been that of strength and superiority that sets its possessor above the rank and file of people" (25). Persons are not of equal worth in the Greek world, nor did Aristotle believe that each person could have a unique or particular function different from others. He was concerned with what set one species apart from another and what set one class of persons above another:

> Elitism is inherent in his whole conception of ethics. The most basic questions of ethics could not even arise for Aristotle if he were required to assume, in the face of all experience, that all persons are inherently or by nature *equal.* It was for the very function of ethics to nourish and increase their inequality, to enable those who are naturally better to rise as far as possible above others with respect to individual worth. Indeed, if we had to suppose that all persons are by nature of equal worth, then what would be the point of talking about human goodness or virtue in the first place? (Taylor 1991, 66).

Aristotle should not be thought of as benighted or ignorant. Living in a hierarchical society seemed "natural" to him and to his fellows. Aristotle believed that the citizen class of men had the capacity to reason better than women, slaves, and those of the lower classes. Reason or rationality was the essential nature of man, and he believed that the men of his class naturally strove to perfect this essence. It was the way of the world—a part of his metaphysics. People of other classes were ruled by their passions and appetites and therefore were essentially slaves or more closely related to animals—unable to control their desires using reason. Thus, the men of his class were born to rule because they have more rationality and reason is the highest part of the soul, whereas the passions, emotions, and desires were "lower" and in need of control.

Doubts about Virtue Ethics

Today we say that all persons are equal in that they have "equal moral worth." Whether they reason well or not, at some fundamental level some things may not be done to them. We accord this equality to babies, the retarded, the insane, the comatose, and the senile who do not reason at all. Why do we do that? As discussed in a section above, some philosophers such as Regan and Singer have suggested that being the "subject-of-a-life" is the criterion for granting moral worth to any being. All "subjects" are the equal of every other. The difficulties with that criterion have been reviewed above. But, in order to incorporate the modern notion of equal worth into virtue ethics, some conception of human nature other than simply being a living subject is needed. Because character traits are basic, and babies, the insane and others may not have any virtues at all, what could be the basis for saying everyone is equal? One might hold that each person has the capacity for attaining virtue and so is equal. So in the *end* we are all equal. One can only have a virtue against the background of understanding what kind of person one should aim to be. That, in turn, probably requires an essentialist notion of human nature. Humans have a fixed essence; it can be understood; and we should aim for it if we are to be good persons.

Along those lines, many philosophers argue that this kind of teleological understanding of human nature is necessary for any adequate virtue ethics (see MacIntyre 1984; Kultgen 1998a,b; and others). An essentialist understanding allows someone to become a better person by linking her present character with some more ideal person she might become if she were to fulfill herself more completely (203–25). Such a teleological understanding may be available within theological systems where God's intentions for human beings are revealed through commandments and doctrine. In a philosophical system that does not rely on religion, arguing for such an essence of human being tends to rely on observation of what men do and what women do. But we all know that roles have changed dramatically over time as women have been permitted more and more access to education and opportunity. Is there any essential "masculine" nature or any essential "feminine" nature? In my view, the preponderance of empirical evidence suggests that some obvious differences are real but that does not justify a belief in essentialism. Human beings have almost limitless capacities for assuming any number and variety of social roles. So, then, could we dispense with essentialism and keep an egalitarian virtue ethics?

Hoping to avoid the necessity of positing an ideal human nature, Edmund Pincoffs (1986) proposes a "nonteleological functionalist" ethics of virtue. That is, each person's life can be morally good without having to aim at anything beyond one's own personal "flourishing." No ideal human nature need be posited. Each person can seek the good in her own personal way and develop as a unique individual. She will, to be sure, seek to flourish as a member of her society and to live a moral life within it. So, if her search is sincere, she seems likely to achieve a good and virtuous life. And as long as she accepts the idea that equality is built upon each person being able to practice this kind of personal quest and change directions if she finds herself on an evil track, then it would appear that the divide between equality and nonessentialism is bridged. Or is it?

Pincoffs' view has been challenged as mere "values clarification" that limits "moral reflection . . . to tracing out a 'pattern of the moral life' while merely assuming the truth of all those other considerations which render the pattern defensible" (Hittinger 1989, 453; see also MacIntyre 1988). That is, the pattern of anyone's flourishing or "healthy personhood" has no defense beyond her own personal taste. Hittinger (1989) also points out that without a teleological understanding of human excellence the person has no way to conceive of herself as a unity: actions stand as piecemeal parts of her character without a harmonious pattern. One's character just becomes whatever one has chosen in light of the values one already has or decides to adopt along the way. Such choices cannot intelligibly be called "moral" even though they can be called subjectively "good." Thus, to make sense of virtue ethics, one either relies on some pre-established understanding of human nature or the whole process of trying to achieve virtue proceeds from unreflective self-affirmation that provides values clarification but no moral guidance. Virtue ethics collapses to an objectionable aestheticism either way.

More problematic yet, in my view, is "the conflation of character traits with psychological traits" (Tong 1993). Most virtue ethicists today rely heavily on Aristotle's explication of virtue ethics. Aristotle argued for two kinds of virtue: intellectual and moral. Remember from the summary above that intellectual virtues are taught, and according to Aristotle the reason to praise someone with this kind of virtue is that he has been taught to *see* what will make him happy. Those who are able to *perform* the moral virtues are praiseworthy simply because they can, in fact, do the action (Tong 1993). Our "list of moral virtues tends to be more restricted than Aristotle's, whose scheme includes courage, temperance, liberality, magnificence, pride, ambition, good temper, friendliness, truthfulness, ready wit, shame, and justice" (Tong 1993, 28). But should it matter in the consideration of his prison sentence whether a thief can tell a good joke? Ethicists today realize that making yourself happy, fulfilled, or flourishing may make someone else unhappy, unfulfilled, or deteriorated. That means that we need to know when we can pursue our personal happiness and when we must set it aside. Moral traits or virtues should permit us to do the right thing. The remaining traits, while good, must be nonmoral. That is, nonmoral traits make you a likeable person, but not a *good* one. Other traits, such as courage and truthfulness, are characteristics of all good persons (Tong 1993).

Various cultures have praised different virtues over time, and invariably many virtues have been gender-specific. For example, the Greek heroic warrior on the battlefield was the example to be emulated for the virtue of courage. According to Aristotle, men show courage by commanding, whereas women show courage by obeying (Bell 1983). Aristotle believed that men had an essentially different and superior human nature to that of women. Thus, the sexes had separate virtues. Many character traits remain gendered in conventional conceptions of our society (for instance, women should be patient, men should be bold). The question is, which of these traits are moral and which are nonmoral? Tong suggests that one may distinguish a moral virtue from a nonmoral one by the fact that "moral virtues are more directly tied to *ungendered character traits* (traits that any person, male or female, has to cultivate in order to be regarded as a good person). Another criterion links moral virtues more closely to recognized moral principles and sets the nonmoral traits aside as desirable but unrelated to morality. That is, a courageous person is no less morally good for being humorless. Nonmoral character traits are often gendered. That is, in order to be considered "feminine" a woman must cultivate traits such as "gentleness, modesty, humility, supportiveness, empathy, compassion, tenderness, nurturance, intuitiveness, sensitivity, and unselfishness" (Tong 1993, 30). To be considered "masculine," one must cultivate traits such as "strength of will, ambition, courage, independence, assertiveness, hardiness, rationality, and emotional control . . . as well as a few distinctively human moral virtues: honesty and justice, to name two" (29). Professor Tong names these traits and virtues in the context of explaining the *virtues* enumerated for men and women of the eighteenth and nineteenth century, when no distinction was made between moral and nonmoral virtues. (It is astonishing to look over the list and think about my undergraduates—how tenacious these genderings remain, even if some progress has been made!) Professor Tong also notes that in that era male "virtues" were favored over allegedly female ones.

Because most eighteenth and nineteenth century philosophers did not distinguish social acceptability from moral goodness and all of the virtues were thought to be gendered to fit the different essential natures of men and women, equal rights for women was a matter of hot debate. Many people then, as now, thought that these "virtues," while learned, were *natural* to each sex.

VEGETARIANISM AND VIRTUE

In this section I show why vegetarianism has an affinity with essentialist notions of human being. Some influential people in the nineteenth century and some youth in the twentieth considered vegetarianism more natural, and "natural" action promotes *purity*, it was believed. But I will show why vegetarianism when justified by a notion of purity is actually praising a nonmoral character trait, rather than a moral virtue. I will also include a rather large amount of material on this movement for its usefulness in later chapters showing its similarity with contemporary feminist vegetarians.

In the nineteenth century, vegetarian movements arose in England and the United States. In fact, America's most prominent spiritual vegetarian movement began in the late 1800s with the Seventh-Day Adventist Church. The Kellogg brothers at the more secular Battle Creek Sanatorium had close ties to the church founders and promoted vegetarian diets as healthful (Carson 1957). The English and American movements were both secular and religious in character, but they shared a common appeal to the virtue of *purity*. Purity as vegetarianism was associated with ideals of health, true human nature as naturalness, reality as Mother nature, and with life itself. The vegetarian of the nineteenth century sought the unification of body and soul and of himself with the natural world (Twigg 1979). The central concern of the exhortations to vegetarianism was for the human individual himself, his personal health, his own nature, and his functional unity. In the 1960s through the 1970s, the idea of food purity became *symbolically* associated with the virtue of justice in the civil rights movement of the time. The color of food (whether it was lighter or darker) and the process of its production (processed or organic) had meaning for certain groups even though consuming or abstaining from consuming the foods had no actual effect on whether one's actions were just (Belasco 1989).

Vegetarian ideals of the nineteenth century are documented in a large variety of vegetarian periodicals of the time. Julia Twigg (1979) researched the writings of English vegetarian societies of the late nineteenth century and the 1970s. She shows that vegetarianism arose in a spiritual movement founded on an "ethic of naturalness" where only vegetarian food is seen as "pure." Vegetarians, then and in the 1970s, regarded their food practice as the only pure way of life. Twigg unravels the moral psychology of vegetarian purity:

> wholeness, natural, pure, goodness. . . . Such words play a key role, slipping over from one context to another, linking and validating, underwriting and building up congruences at different levels. Take for example "wholeness." Whole food is food that contains the whole grain. But the word is imbued with much more. Associated within the vegetarian milieu are also ideas of psychic wholeness. There are the associations with holistic medicine which aims to treat the whole body . . . or the whole body and spirit (with all the ideas of the unity of mind and body and the role of the psychological in physical ailments and characteristics that that implies). In their ecological interests . . . we find it crowned in ideas of the unity of all living creatures (central in arguments concerning the evil of inflicting suffering on animals); and above all in the cosmic union of man and nature, and in the belief that the summation of religion and philosophy lies in holism and immanence" (14–15).

In vegetarian ideology, nature becomes "moralized" because vegetarians equate naturalness with goodness, and nature in its underlying *reality* is equated with harmony, pantheistic unity, and redemptive power. Twigg (1979) argues that the central vegetarian theme of "nature and the natural" provide underlying structure and unity for all the other major concerns of vegetarians, most of which are mentioned in the quotation above.[18] I shall be arguing in chapter 7 that this latter association with egalitarianism is misguided.

Twigg also notes that "while there are, analytically, two major strands in the vegetarian argument, stemming either from the rejection of cruelty to animals, or from ideas of health, it is in fact rare to find a vegetarian who would support only one aspect" (16). The relationship to nature, to animals, and the self are intertwined. In looking at the meaning of eating meat, she notes that meat has enjoyed the highest status among foods, and blood carries the focussing imagery in a culture of vitality and power. "Part of the central meaning of red meat is sexuality: meat as flesh, as the flesh, as fleshy delights, as carnality" (17). Blood was thought to carry the particular essence of the person or the animal. For just these reasons it comes closest to the taboo: "that which is most sacred, most highly prized, can by virtue of the strength of its power be the most defiling . . . a peculiarly polluting substance . . . a symbol of . . . crime" (17). Vegetarian revulsion is particularly directed against "red meat—steak dripping with blood" (17). Thus, in eating an animal humans take in the animal's nature and encounter their own animal nature.

A Cartesian dualistic metaphysics pervades the writings. From the sermons in the *Vegetarian Messenger* in 1850, Twigg finds the dualistic love and fear "that the ingestion of animals will break down the constructed barrier between men and the beasts":

> "If . . . we wish to become carniverous [*sic*], ferocious and unclean in our dispositions, practices and desires let us, by all means, follow the dietetic example of those animals which are carniverous, ferocious and unclean" (quoted in Twigg 1979, 20).

In the Western tradition since the time of the Pythagoreans, flesh has been reviled as representative of one's "lower bodily nature" as opposed to the "higher" rational, spiritual, and moral soul. Vegetarianism allowed attainment of the higher virtues by means of controlling, reducing and even eliminating the bodily passions. Thus, the most *real* nature of human beings is not the body and its destructive hungers. Cruelty and aggression are not natural to human beings but are brought on "by a distorting society and a distorted way of eating—the carnivorous" (Twigg 1979, 21). Thus, nonviolence would be an expression of a more natural, spiritual, real humanity.

Vegetarians seek a way of resolving the dualities that appear in the mental/physical, rational/passionate, good/evil dichotomies of everyday life. By identifying human nature as essentially good and nature itself as harmonious and beneficent while society is the evil, the human quest for goodness and moral virtue becomes identified with harmonizing the self with nature. Contact with nature is a source of redemptive power and salvation. Twigg notes that the interest in gardening, rural living, herbalism, dowsing, astrology and other efforts to read the Book of Nature ties in with vegetarian counterculture in the nineteenth century and in the 1970s. The vision of "nature red in tooth and claw" where the living world is understood to persist by life forms feeding upon one another in a "vast canvas of death and predation" is rejected as unreal (22).

Yet, another dichotomy presents itself—humans are at once animals and not animals. Humans are capable of a moral sense that permits them to reflect upon life and death and to transcend animality. It is this moral sense that makes human nature good rather than evil, and yet it is the body and its animality that makes us natural—and it is nature rather than culture that is good. In Twigg's assessment, vegetarians project the picture of harmonized nature back onto humanity and then use that projected picture to criticize society as false, "artificial, inauthentic and distorting" (22). "Society and its manners are . . . something imposed on individuals and not seen as having any positive creative influence on them . . . social structure is identified with divisiveness and exploitation" (27). Only the *"pre-social"* self is natural and good. Similarly, in the 1970s Warren Belasco (1989) finds food concerns linked to class struggle, racial and ethnic equality, unease over the growing complexity, alienation, and fast pace of American life, mistrust of government, capitalism, consumerism, and the media.

Twigg notes connections to the natural in vegetarian preferences for raw fruits and vegetables. Meat must be cooked and cooking is civilized, but vegetarian food can be picked off the trees or out of the ground. The symbolism here is that "nature is . . . superior to culture" (23). What the vegetarian most often does not realize is that in nature we see only ourselves: "Man projects his aspirations out on to nature, and then uses it to judge and condemn society" (23). Twigg (1979) describes an essential reversal of values. Whereas refinement, artistry, and polish had been the purest marks of human excellence (particularly during the Renaissance and Enlightenment), the vegetarian counterculture praises the raw and the "whole natural" in both food and artifacts—raw sugar becomes purer than white sugar, not because other substances (impurities) are absent or the sugar is "unsullied," but because it is closer to the cane. Although the very concept of purity seems inverted, Twigg argues that the "rejection of meat forms a boundary around the pure, within which the ethic of wholeness is unassailed" (23). Meat is impure because of its symbolic association with death and civilization, but junk foods are impure because they are *unreal*, "false, dena-tured, reconstituted, coloured, flavoured and emulsified" (24). Drawing from the macrobiotic journal *Seed*, published from 1971–1977, Twigg reports that junk foods are identified with food, mass culture, consumerism, and thus con-tribute to the alienation of the self. "Trash foods are pre-digested, pappy, super-whippy—food for a slave culture" (24). Only the natural and the living are pure and real and free. Belasco (1989) finds some similar themes in his analysis of the American counterculture's challenge to the food industry in the late 1960s through the late 1970s, although his study shows a symbolic connection to concern with social justice. Belasco documents the anti-establishment, civil rights political overtones in the movement's endorsement of unrefined, "brown" foods and disdain for "white" foods: "Whiteness meant Wonder Bread, White Tower, Cool Whip, Minute Rice, instant mashed potatoes, peeled apples, White Tornadoes, white coats, white collar, whitewash, White House, white racism. Brown meant whole wheat bread, unhulled rice, turbinado sugar, wildflower honey, unsulfured molasses, soy sauce, peasant yams, 'black is beautiful.' Dark-ness was funky, earthy, authentic, while whiteness, the color of powerful deter-gents, suggested fear of contamination and disorder" (48).

The vegetarian movement also reverses the normal usage of the words "alive" and "dead." Vegetarian food is described as vibrant and "alive as the universe is alive . . . filled with the same life as the trees, the plants, the waving grain" (25). Meat is dead. Eating meat is "eating corpses . . . the ingestion of dead animals is an ingestion of death itself" (25). Symbolically, vegetarianism rejects death and in so doing offers a "this-worldly" salvation of the body, imaging the re-establishment of Eden where the dichotomies of life are resolved into a state of natural harmony. Twigg emphasizes that the tradition attempts to be anti-Cartesian and the spirit and life that are valued in vegetarian food are of this world: "it is a spiritual body that is being stressed, not a disembodied spirit" (26).

The pure body is alive with feeling and intensity of expression. Vegetarian "anxiety about eating . . . relates to this image of the pure body. There is a fear of taking into the body something nasty or impure. . . . At times even the processes of digestion are seen as alien,.. so that the body under total fast is restored to a pure state. . . . What vegetarianism presents therefore is a risen, Blakean picture of the body, an immortal, youthful temple of the spirit" (26–27).

Twigg (1979) notes the recurrence of themes of salvation, renewal, purity, health, and social reform in vegetarian culture. Vegetarianism "has been associated with all the major reform movements from anti-slavery, pacifism, penal reform, women's rights, CND, and with most of the major utopias, underpinning attempts to create the New Age from Owenism, to Whiteway, to the Aquarian Age . . . It is this capacity to act as a condensed and unifying symbol, drawing together the different levels of experience, that causes vegetarianism to flourish in periods and among groups where holistic answers are sought" (29, 31). Belasco (1989) notes the association of vegetarianism with the environmental movement. Frances Moore Lappé's *Diet for a Small Planet* (1971) "soon became *the* vegetarian text of the ecology movement" (56). The appeal was to the wastefulness of the meat-centered diet. Gary Snyder's philosophy of "living lightly" swirled together with Robert Rodale's prescriptions for organic gardening and farming and myriad other forces to produce a resurgence of interest in "naturalness" and "wholeness" in food, although not always vegetarian cuisine, that had been a common theme in nineteenth-century vegetarian philosophy.

Vegetarianism presents itself as signaling the coming of a New Moral Order. And yet its ethic of naturalness and ontology of unity make it impossible to understand the suffering, violence, social strife, human vanity, war, cruelty, and death that are a part of our everyday experience. The vegetarian ideology extracts the evil away, defining it as *unreality* and placing it outside of the system. What remains is good and pure, alive and safe. That and that alone is natural. The new ethics of naturalness and purity affirms egalitarianism and looks to overturn the old social order by abolishing social structure and re-establishing an ideal pre-social harmony where the lion lies down with the lamb.

In sum, virtue ethics differs from rule-based ethics in asserting that moral character is primary and that judgments of virtue can be made apart from judgments about actions. The identification of the "natural" with the "good" dates back at least to the Greeks. Aristotle thought one must have both intellectual and moral virtue in order to achieve fulfillment in accordance with one's unique essence as human. Today, virtue ethicists realize that some traits, such as wit and magnificence, are desirable because they are socially advantageous to the bearer, whereas others are desirable whether or not they benefit the bearer. Thus, some traits commonly referred to as virtues are better referred to as nonmoral traits, or as I shall refer to the one associated with vegetarianism, an aesthetic preference-trait. Some vegetarians have incorporated the supposed virtue of purity into a naturalistic ethics that defines or abstracts away all evils from pre-social human nature. Disharmony, cruelty, suffering, and death are unnatural. Pre-social humans are equally natural and good. No reasons are given for these foundational beliefs, and in some aspects these beliefs are inconsistent and are projections of human fears. The reasons given to practice vegetarianism differ from those offered by Regan, Singer, and others in the duty-based ethical tradition. The primary virtue-based reasons offered to practice a vegetarian diet are to find harmony, unity, and self-fulfillment. Such a "virtue" is better described as a nonmoral psychological or aesthetic preference-trait.

The next chapter discusses contemporary feminist ethical vegetarianism, both for its similarities and differences from the traditional duty-based theories. Even though virtually all of these writers eschew traditional rule-based moral theory, many of their arguments and approaches appear to assume most of its concepts and structure. Others move toward a virtue ethics that endorses dispositions and attitudes that function as virtues. But, as I will show, neither traditional moral theory nor feminist ethics can successfully argue for ethical vegetarianism and still maintain their foundational principles or beliefs.

CHAPTER 3

FEMINISM AND ETHICAL VEGETARIANISM

Feminism, vegetarianism, and moral concern for animals have historical connections. Many nineteenth-century English and American feminists were antivivisectionists and vegetarians. In 1875, Frances Power Cobbe co-founded the Victoria Street Society for the Protection of Animals Liable to Vivisection (VSS) and later the British Union for the Abolition of Vivisection (BUAV) (Elston 1987). The list of such "first-wave" feminists who wrote, spoke, or worked in support of the cause of animals or advocated vegetarianism is long: In a 1990 article, Josephine Donovan lists Mary Wollstonecraft, Harriet Beecher Stowe, Lydia Maria Child, Elizabeth Blackwell, Elizabeth Stuart Phelps Ward, Susan B. Anthony, Victoria Woodhull, Elizabeth Cady Stanton, the Grimké sisters, Lucy Stone, Frances Willard, Anna Kingsford, Caroline Earle White, Margaret Fuller, Charlotte Perkins Gilman, and Agnes Ryan (359). In addition, Mary Ann Elston (1987) identifies many other women antivivisectionists—some of them, like Cobbe, who were not vegetarians—and some of whom, like Queen Victoria, could not be classified as feminists.[1] Likewise, the physician and Theosophist Anna Kingsford was an especially influential crusader against vivisection and meat eating (Elston 1987). Margaret Fuller opposed the slaughter of animals for food in *Woman of the Nineteenth Century* (1845) and argued that liberating women into public life would transform male-dominated violent society into a vegetarian culture of "plant-like gentleness" (Donovan 1990).[2] Frances Willard "believed flesh-eating was 'savagery' and that the 'enlightened mortals of the twentieth century [would] surely be vegetarians'" (quoted in Donovan 1990, 359, n. 29). In their idealized vegetarian future, Fuller, Willard and other early feminist vegetarians perhaps subscribed to the beliefs discussed in Twigg's (1979) article. And they believed well-balanced vegetarian diets to be as healthful as omnivorous diets.[3]

Most early feminists who opposed experimentation on live animals, hunting, trapping, and raising animals for food based their activism on sensitivity to the sufferings of animals, a different kind of reason than Twigg discusses. For example, Charlotte Perkins Gilman condemned trapping and the wearing of fur: "Trapping means every agony known to an animal, imprisonment, starvation, freezing, frantic fear and pain. If one woman hung up or fastened down hundreds of kittens each by one paw in her backyard in winter weather, to struggle and dangle and freeze, to cry in anguish and terror that she might 'trim' something with their collected skins . . . she would be considered a monster" (quoted in Donovan 1990, 352–53). Gilman's arguments, though, are apparently based in a proscription against cruelty, rather than any notion of the equality of animals. Gilman envisions a vegetarian society in her utopian *Herland* (1915), but her ideal society excludes domesticated food animals altogether:

> As to the wild beasts—there were none in their sheltered land. . . .
>
> "Have you no cattle—sheep—horses?" . . .
>
> "We had, in the very old days, . . ."
>
> "What became of them? . . . "
>
> "We do not want them anymore. They took up too much room—we need all our land to feed our people. It is such a little country, you know" (49).

Humans were still seen as more important than animals, and animals appear to be expendable to a human community. Feminist alliances for stringent equality for animals would not emerge in earnest for sixty more years.

Although the humane movement continued at a low key in the United States and Europe, its specific association with feminism did not reappear in the United States until the mid-1970s, when Carol Adams published two articles linking feminism and vegetarianism (1975, 1976). At the same time, Peter Singer published *Animal Liberation* (1975). By the early 1980s, Constantia Salamone (1982) published her article on women and animal rights, and Bernard Rollin (1981) and Tom Regan (1983) had published their books using traditional moral rights theory to argue that animals are members of the moral community with equal rights. A large number of journal articles and books cascaded in the aftermath of these early writings.[4] The vast majority of these argued from the traditional moral theories that formed the body of philosophical thought about ethics at the time.

RECENT FEMINIST CRITICISMS OF
THE RULE-BASED TRADITION

Contemporary feminists have critiqued traditional moral theory on a variety of fronts, and many lively debates are going on in the philosophical and feminist literature. I shall not be able to discuss all of the strands of these arguments in detail. Instead, I will give some explanations of the variety of approaches with emphasis on those making significant comment concerning animal welfare and vegetarianism.

ETHICS OF CARE

Most feminist writers who defend ethical vegetarianism claim to use an ethics of care as the basis for their arguments. Perhaps the most famous of care theorists is Carol Gilligan, who in 1977 and later in her 1982 book challenged then-current theories of moral development. Using her own studies, Gilligan challenged the assumptions in Lawrence Kohlberg's six-level scale of moral development (Kohlberg 1969; Kohlberg and Kramer 1969). On his scale the least morally mature people base their decisions on the needs of the self. People who use universal principles based on abstract, objective rationality attain the last, sixth (and thus, highest or best) stage of moral development. On testing Kohlberg (1971) discovered most men reach stage five, but he found a "strong interpersonal bias" in many of the women he tested, placing them at about stage three, a level of "interpersonal concordance." At this stage, people choose their ethical actions, not because of some universal rule about right behavior, but because "the good is identified with 'what pleases or helps others and is approved by them'" (Gilligan 1977, 484, quoting Kohlberg 1971).

Women appeared to be morally stunted on Kohlberg's assessment scale and largely incapable of thinking about moral issues in terms of abstraction.[5] But why accept the idea that acting on abstract moral principles signals the highest stage of moral development? That assumption is an arbitrary one based on a scale made up by Kohlberg. Gilligan suspected that Kohlberg's original study (and others before it) had been biased by its exclusion of girls and women and a preference for a "male voice," so she conducted a study of females (Gilligan

1977, 1982). From her study, she argued that girls and boys solve ethical problems in different ways. Whereas boys and young men learn very early to appeal to rules and rights to decide about conflicting interests, girls and young women exhibit sensitivity to the feelings of others and prefer to use the notions of caring and responsibility as moral categories. Boys use rules to allow a game to continue, and sometimes that results in excluding someone from playing. Girls will abandon the game rather than break up the group. Later in their development, she claimed, women look at an ethical problem in the context of preserving relationships, community, family, and friendships and are willing to sacrifice their own good to assure that others are not harmed. The most morally mature women, on Gilligan's new scale, see that they themselves have value, that self-sacrifice has some limits, and that no one should be harmed. Gilligan identifies the morality of nonviolence as the last (and thus, highest or best) level of women's moral development, a level that can be achieved by any person nevertheless. Women, therefore, "speak in a different voice" from their male counterparts. But their moral contribution to culture is no less important. Nor is their moral conceptualizing completely devoid of abstraction. Gilligan notes that women do emphasize concrete, personal contexts, but the morality of nonviolence is a stage which admits abstraction and universality in its aims that no one be harmed. Philosophers note, too, that Kohlberg's scale parallels the scale of esteem for rational justification that appears in the philosophical literature on traditional moral theory. Egocentric reasons are least acceptable and fear of punishment is contemptible, whereas appeal to rules of justice is most enlightened. Neither Kohlberg's nor Gilligan's study is value-free, although Kohlberg's reflects dominant conventional ideas of the right and the good to a greater degree.

Gilligan delineated some important moral categories which are alive in our culture but have been neglected or omitted from moral psychology and philosophy. Whereas rule-driven, relatively impersonal and universal *justice* is the basis of morality for male-dominated culture, many women tend to assess morality from the perspective of *caring* about people in relationships and in the particularity of their situations or context. Women realize that relationships of the family and community are not contracts among equals, but are ethical ties bound by joy and pain and the fundamentally caring nature of humans.

Gilligan's work has been attacked on probably over a dozen fronts, most of which I shall not be able to outline here (see Tong 1993 for a review). The most important general criticism for our purposes concerns the division of justice from care and their division along gendered lines. If two "separate-but-equal" voices exist, then men and women cannot help but talk past each other in discussions of ethics. The difference in voice may continue rather than relieve the oppression of women and those men who are not of the dominant class. Because caring apparently permits obligation only if the people are in a close relationship, would impartial justice go out the window in a revised ethics? The resolution of impartial justice with caring has been a major project of feminist ethicists, and in her later writings Gilligan has attempted to clarify and develop her views (Gilligan 1995): "listening to women's voices clarified the ethic of care, not because care is essentially associated with women or part of women's nature, but because women for a combination of psychological and political reasons voiced relational realities that were otherwise unspoken or dismissed as inconsequential" (1995, 123). Thus, the voice is not tied specifically to women. Gilligan has "theorized both justice and care in relational terms. Justice speaks to the disconnections which are at the root of violence, violation and oppression, or the unjust use of unequal power. Care speaks to the dissociations which lead people to abandon themselves and others. . . . The antidote to psychological repression is the antidote to totalitarianism" (1995, 125).

A second important criticism is related to the above: in attributing an ethic of care to women Gilligan reinforces the idea that women are born in a certain way and have a biologically determined nature. Cressida Heyes (1997) examines anti-essentialist claims about Gilligan's work and argues that Gilligan's recent research requires that these charges be rethought. I will discuss essentialism and nonessentialism later in this book.

RELATIONAL FEMININE ETHICS OF CARING

A second important notion of care is explicated in Nel Noddings' *Caring: A Feminine Approach to Ethics and Moral Education* (1984). Noddings claims that her view expresses an *alternative voice* which is better than traditional moral theories of justice, whereas Gilligan argued that justice and care are compatible equals. Noddings argues that ethics is based on one-on-one relationships of caring. These she calls the relationship of the "one-caring" and the "one-cared-for." The one-cared-for and the one-caring maintain the ethical relationship through a subjective experience of receptivity, relatedness, and responsiveness. The beginning of an ethical life arises from the emotional desire to become a good person. This, in turn, has arisen from the desire to "preserve our deepest and most tender human feelings. The caring of mother for child, of human adult for human infant. . . . For many women, this feeling of nurturance is at the very heart of what we assess as good" (Noddings 1984, 87) While rational analysis has a place in her theory, she continuously argues that such analysis is not helpful to moral teaching. Emotions and feelings are much more important.

Feeling and caring are always centered on those one knows personally, and not towards those with whom we have no connection. Does she mean that no one has any obligation to those unknown? Noddings says that we are all connected by "chains" of caring that permit us to care more for our own family members and still feel and act on a desire to help those far away from and unknown to us. The one-caring and one-cared-for relationship is supposed to be mutual, responsive, reciprocal, and therefore equal. For those close to us but for whom we are not particularly disposed to care, Noddings brings in the criterion of *potential relation* (1984, 87). That is, if the one-cared-for has a potentiality to respond in a dynamic relationship, then "we must meet that other as one-caring" (1984, 86). Thus, Noddings believes that humans have responsibilities to unborn fetuses after the second trimester because of this potential for relationship, for example.

Unlike Gilligan, Noddings specifically mentions obligations to animals. She believes that we do not have direct obligations to them. Why? "The potential of animals . . . is nearly static; they cannot respond in mutuality, nor can the nature of their response change substantially" (87). Although I think her attitude about animals suggests that she may not know animals very well, I do agree with her comment as follows: "A philosophical position that has difficulty distinguishing between our obligation to human infants and, say, pigs is in some difficulty straight off" (87).

Noddings' work has been criticized on several fronts, especially for its focus on relationships of unequal power and dependency as the paradigm of ethics. Similarly, her focus on intimate relationships seems to make obligations to strangers problematic. And her focus on the one-cared-for as the center of the moral point-of-view brings women to the point of exploitation. Critics charge that the *feminine* ethics valorizes self-sacrifice to the brink of self-abuse and destruction, certainly an ethics *feminists* would not wish to adopt (see Card 1990; Hoagland 1990; Houston 1990; and Noddings 1990). I shall not have time or space to discuss the merits of Noddings' views or those of her critics. But it is immediately apparent that several views of an ethics of care are possible.

For example, Gilligan (1995) distinguishes her view sharply from a *feminine* ethics. She maintains that "a feminine ethic of care is an ethic of the relational world as that world appears within a patriarchal social order: that is, as a world apart, separated politically and psychologically from a realm of individual autonomy and freedom which is the realm of justice and contractual obligation" (122). The patriarchal judgment may valorize disconnection, calling it autonomy, independence, self-determination, what you will. But, a *feminist* ethic of care, she argues, is founded on connection, and this experience of connection is not "unnatural, unhealthy, or unreal" (121). The challenge is to learn "how to listen to women in women's terms, rather than assimilating women's voices to the existing theoretical framework" (120).

MATERNAL ETHICS

Virginia Held (1993) and Sara Ruddick (1989) have written extensively on mothering and maternal thinking as foundational to ethical thinking. Love, nurturance, protection, and preservation of mothers or any person who is mothering is the moral experience that is the primary model for ethics. Critics charge that these frameworks idealize mothering too much, exclude men, and ignore the differences among mothers. A fuller discussion of maternal ethics and of whether or not these criticisms are justifiable would take us too far afield at the moment.

CARE OR JUSTICE?

Held (1995) has joined several other thinkers in attempting to work out one of the major difficulties facing an ethics of care: how to reconcile care with justice and impartiality. Justice requires impartiality, but care requires partiality. Helga Kuhse, Peter Singer, and Maurice Rickard (1998) have recently discussed the problems of sameness and difference, partiality and impartiality, among women and men. They point out that "the different feminist views within the sameness theme are all likely to share a very general commitment to justice, universality, equal respect and treatment, and allocation of benefits and burdens according to *merit*" (Kushse *et al.* 1998, 455–56, emphasis added). These expectations call upon impartial justice and a demand for the *same* treatment. Kuhse *et al.* (1998) claim that "the issue we now confront is that of how the idea of a partialist ethic for women shapes up in the context of certain impartialist concerns" (456). For example, hiring should be done without concern for a caring relation to the hired.

More generally, the problem is, how does difference fit into the existing system of equality as sameness? Joy Kroeger-Mappes (1994), in concert with a great many other feminist thinkers, argues that the ethic of rights, which Kuhse *et al.* (1998) call the impartialist ethic, and the ethic of care are both part of the same faulty system. On Kroeger-Mappes' view the ethic of care is the basis for the ethics of rights. Held (1995) echoes this, saying that "care should be the wider moral framework into which justice should be fitted" (128). Traditional rights theories depend upon atomistic conceptions of the self and freedom. In order to develop the idea that care is the basis of rights, Diana Tietjens Meyers (1989, 1993) proposes a relational model of self and autonomy. She claims that an ethic of care does not require Kantian theoretical commitments. Rather than being individualistic, autonomy can be "made possible by our social relations" (157) and that skills for autonomy are gained through social training, wherein people learn to monitor their own conduct in relationship to others. Jean Keller (1997) uses Meyers' theory to propose "a dialogical model of autonomy . . . that can respond to internal and external critiques of care ethics" (152). The question of whether we ought to consider care or justice fundamental is an ongoing topic of debate in feminist scholarship. Here we see Kuhse, Singer, and Rickard placing impartiality first, and in a later section I will show that Tom Regan proceeds in the same manner. In these short sections I have given brief summaries of the issues in order to set the context for my own claims about a much narrower concern, that of ethical vegetarianism. In what follows I will be confining my discussion primarily to ecofeminists who have argued for ethical vegetarianism. All of them have claimed the basis of their views as an ethics of care.

OTHER FEATURES OF FEMINIST ETHICS OF CARE

Contextualism

Most feminists who argue for an ethics of care claim that their ethics is also a "contextual ethics." A contextual ethic applies within some contexts and not others. It avoids appeal to universal rules. Nevertheless, each situation must be evaluated in its particularity and richness of context. An action which seemed right in one context may be wrong in others. Feminist contextualists claim that the approach differs from the traditional (*ala* Regan 1983) in that "the rights approach is not inherently contextual (it is the response to the rights of all sentient beings), [whereas] the caring-for approach responds to particular contexts and histories. It recognizes that the reasons for moral vegetarianism may differ by locale, by gender, as well as by class" (Curtin 1991, 68–69). Nevertheless, context evaluation is essential to traditional rule-centered ethics, act-utilitarianism, and virtue ethics. Modern traditionalists reject blind obedience to absolute rules and readily admit that the right rule or action to take varies with the context or situation. Evaluation within context is not unique to feminist contextualist views. But, feminists emphasize the *richness* of the contexts. Every situation differs from every single other one.

Placing too great an emphasis on context can create some problems. If contextualists were to insist on the extreme differences among contexts, then no previous situation would serve as any kind of guide to the next situation. Each would appear anew. Past cases would be irrelevant to present ones. No rules could be developed, and even experience itself might be of little value in attempting to decide what to do in any particular case. Although many writers in feminist ethics reject the value of rules in ethics, few reject experience. At least some comparison of the past with the present and future seems essential to ethical action. Having commitments and beliefs about what makes some situations similar to others establishes the basis for logical and moral consistency. If one were to approach each context completely anew, then one's decisions would more likely be based on the mood of the moment, prejudices, whim, and so forth. Without some reference to criteria of similarity, one's decisions become arbitrary and morally inconsistent. But arbitrariness and inconsistency are morally vicious— that is, unjust, uncaring, unfair. So, feminist contextualists must agree that some comparisons among contexts are appropriate. Rules-of-thumb might be appropriately applied.

If some comparisons among contexts are appropriate, then moral contextualists should agree that certain categories of contexts exist where the cases within them loosely resemble one another. For moral decision making, one must embroider the context sufficiently in order to see how the present context might overlap those of many kinds of past contexts that she has experienced or has been taught to recognize from the experience of others.

POLITICIZING ETHICS

Because traditional rule-based ethics and ethical theory can be used as a club to subordinate women (see Sherwin 1989 and Littleton 1987), feminists argue that ethics must be "politicized." Politicizing ethics means that people must recognize that the genders are differently situated with respect to actual power today. A politicized ethic would consider right and wrong, virtue and vice, by recognizing the inequality of existing power structures. Women and men remain unequal, and society and its institutions presuppose and expect that inequality. Any attempt at neutralized application of the rules will only further serve the class in power. No ideal or applied ethic can be fair unless it takes account of the fact that some groups have less voice or no voice at all.

PLURALISM OF NORMS

Those arguing for an ethics of care also claim that norms within contexts are *pluralistic*. Even if most people agree on the various good things in life, different people hold different kinds of values as more important than others. But, no objective scale exists against which to decide which of these values is most important in any particular context. Usually, the differences are not about whether a particular value is good, but rather whether it is best or most important in a particular context. For example, in the debate about physician-assisted suicide, those on both sides agree that autonomy or self-determination is generally a good thing. But, on one interpretation, opponents think that self-determination should be limited and should not apply when it comes to choosing the time of one's own death, whereas advocates believe autonomy should not be so restricted.

A choice under pluralism relies on the beliefs of the individual, but no person's beliefs can be shown to be objectively true or false despite a large amount of reasonable argumentation. Yet, the pluralist avoids relativism because decisions that diverge from hers can be *right* or "justified" if the intentions, rules, care, or experience to which others appeal are good in some other contexts and the consequences are not obviously unjust, uncaring, or unfair. Rather than absolute or objective truth, such decisions might be said to offer "fuzzy truth." Given a plurality of norms, rules and virtues cannot be universally applicable across the context boundaries.

While the above review of the ethics of care is brief, I hope that it is sufficient for my purposes. Those who desire a fuller understanding should refer to the references cited. I shall now turn to questions of how those espousing an ethics of care argue that we know that animals should be equal partners in the moral community.

FEMINIST EPISTEMOLOGY AND
THE MORAL STANDING OF ANIMALS

Division has been marked along gender lines about the epistemological basis for obligations to humans and animals. From the first, (mostly male) scientists dismissed feelings, emotions, or sentiment[6] as an adequate basis for animal rights and responded with "rational" arguments that animals were not conscious beings and did not actually suffer pain.[7] In the late nineteenth century, Henry Salt (1892) argued for the rights of animals based on reason as opposed to sentiment. The supposed opposition between reason and emotion has continued to dominate the debate, with mostly male thinkers arguing *for* reason and *against* emotion as an adequate basis for obligations to animals. Included in this partisan polemic are Peter Singer and Tom Regan, who specifically denied that considerations of sentiment and emotion could be adequate foundations for the rights and welfare of animals (see Donovan 1990; see also Singer 1975, 1981, and Regan 1983, 1991).

Some feminists think that a properly construed feminist epistemology and ontology can ground animal rights and ethical vegetarianism.[8] Josephine Donovan (1990, 1996) and Marti Kheel (1985) critique Singer and Regan for rejecting emotion and caring: "Natural rights and utilitarianism present impressive and useful philosophical arguments for the ethical treatment of animals. Yet, it is also possible—indeed, necessary—to ground that ethic in an emotional and spiritual conversation with nonhuman life-forms" (Donovan 1990, 375). Donovan argues that "out of a women's relational culture of caring and attentive love, therefore, emerges the basis for a feminist ethic for the treatment of animals. We should not kill, eat, torture, and exploit animals because they do not want to be so treated, and we know that" (1990, 375). Donovan argues that we know that animals do not wish to be so treated through "an emotional and spiritual conversation" with them (1990, 375). "Such a conversation can emerge only when attentive love is directed at them" (Donovan 1996, 95–96). Donovan draws on a long tradition of sympathy theorists, including David Hume, Arthur Schopenhauer, Martin Buber, Edmund Husserl, Max Scheler, Simone Weil, H. B. Acton, and Iris Murdoch for her claim that the emotions and attentive love, in particular, provide epistemic ground for moral knowledge. Donovan believes that the experience engendered by attentive love will serve as a foundation for feminist ethics and ethical prescriptions. She does express an abolitionism similar to that of Carol Adams, whose work is discussed below.

Following Rosemary Radford Ruether (1975), Sara Ruddick (1989), Paula Gunn Allen (1986) and other feminists, Donovan takes as her primary purpose the cultivation of "ways in which our thinking about animal/human relationships may be reoriented" (374–75). That ethical reorientation "requires a fundamental respect for nonhuman life-forms, an ethic that listens to and accepts the diversity of environmental voices and the validity of their realities, . . . resists wrenching and manipulating the context so as to subdue it to one's categories; it is nonimperialistic and life affirming" (1990, 374). Donovan describes an attitude that one should take to be and become humane. She extols the deep respect people ought to adopt for nature and animals. As she says, "people exercising attentive love *see* the tree, but they also see the logging industry. They see the downed cow in the slaughterhouse pen; but they also see the farming and dairy industry. They see the Silver Spring monkey, but they also see the drug corporations and university collaboration" (1996, 98, italics in original). Donovan and many feminists like her argue for a politicized ethics that focuses on the social institutions and entrenched power structures that influence the lives and choices of individuals.

I agree with Donovan that some form of sentiment and emotion should be recognized in moral epistemology. These passionate assessments coupled with rational judgments about the moral standing of animals give us knowledge of the suffering of humans and animals. That is not being challenged here in this book. Rather, I am pointing to a context that is larger than some feminists, animal rights and welfare advocates, and environmentalists are seeing—that real conflict among the needs and interests of various groups exist. Equality, justice, and caring require that we formulate a decision procedure that will guide us through the maze of these conflicts.

Donovan (1990, 1996) appears to believe that the prescription of moral respect enriched by sympathetic attentive love will generate the morality necessary to abolish the use of animals and ground an ethical vegetarianism. But her argument begs the question. The question is "what does moral respect require of us?" Moral respect is a rather slippery concept—you must already know what it means to respect someone in order to practice it. But if you already know that, then this moral concept is not fundamental and is instead grounded on some more basic moral virtue or imperative. Such a theory becomes originally circular and vulnerable to conventionalism.

Especially in her 1996 article, Donovan is careful to confine her discussion to concerns of moral epistemology. She expresses a belief that the infusion of caring in addition to the arguments from justice and rights will motivate a response in people to care about animals (98). Thus, she appears to believe, as did the ancient Greeks, that all (or at least most) moral error is done in ignorance. When humans discover the truth, they will act rightly. In her 1990 article in a hypothetical choice between a nonhuman animal and a human, she sidesteps the issue, saying that such examples present us with the "either/or" and we should work for the "both/and." While it is always desirable to have more knowledge, conflict abounds in our everyday lives. When the ideal of harmony, peace, co-existence, love, unity, and understanding cannot be realized, Donovan offers no guidance to one who would choose rightly. Donovan's view seems unhelpful because the very "diversity of environmental voices and the validity of their realities" placed in the context of our *mortality* make moral choices in the face of conflict imminent and singular. How will Donovan's abolitionist ethical view help Penny to decide whether to eat beef liver to boost her iron deficient state? or Rachel to decide whether it is morally permissible to feed her children "cold bologna"? Feminists wish to bridge dichotomies, but there is a danger that in so doing we may retreat into abstraction and the idealism of "*if only* everyone cared and had proper reverence, all conflict would be resolved." We must remember even if everyone reasons well and everyone cares, some moral conflict will still exist. I shall argue in chapter 7 that real caring requires far less meat eating but not abstention and need not require ethical vegetarianism.

TOM REGAN'S REJECTION OF FEMINIST EPISTEMOLOGY

REGAN'S ARGUMENT

In his recent book, *The Thee Generation* (1991), Tom Regan devotes a chapter to "Feminism and Vivisection" in which he concludes that an "ethic-of-care feminism" cannot provide an adequate ground for the rights of animals.[9] Regan's argument for this conclusion goes like this: "First-wave" liberal feminism argued for freedoms based on similarities of women and men and embraced the male-dominated world and its values without question. More recently, cultural feminists have challenged the liberal feminist view. The cultural feminists claim that women experience the world in ways that differ from males. Women have made specific and valued contributions to culture. Most white males in Western culture live in positions of power and privilege less open or not open to women. Because of their social roles, women (in general) have developed moral perspectives that are based on relationship and caring. Such attitudes are antithetical to the domination inherent in patriarchy, and therefore feminists must reject all patriarchy. However, in order to reject patriarchy and its domination, feminists must reject assumptions of human distinctness and superiority to nonhuman animals. So, Regan argues that ethic-of-care feminism, in rejecting the liberal feminist view, should see no value distinction between themselves and nonhuman animals. It follows then that ethic-of-care feminists must accept "our *moral equality* with those animals who are otherwise like us . . . who, like us, respond to the world emotionally (through fear and anxiety, for example). Thus, if an enlightened feminist perspective would find it wrong to make a human animal suffer . . . it seems that this same perspective must make the same finding if a nonhuman animal is made to suffer" (Regan 1991, 94). Here, his main point is that ethic-of-care feminists *must accept a principle of equality* if they argue for animal welfare, for vegetarianism, and against vivisection. On this point, Regan is correct.

Regan (1991) then asks whether an ethic-of-care feminism can provide a sufficient ground for the Principle of Equality. His answer is "no." He gives two reasons why caring cannot be an adequate foundation. First, if caring is all that matters or what matters most, then what we do for others depends "entirely on *how much one cares* for these individuals" (95). Regan then objects that this is a "'chancy' basis" for morality: "The very bonds of caring that unite us with some, divide us from others" (95). Regan bases his objection on the idea of *impartiality*, which he states operationally: "To judge impartially is not to allow any personal factor to prejudice one's judgment" (86). Caring about individual persons can prejudice our judgments, in his view, and thus lead us into injustice. Labeling this view a "moral conservatism," he notes that people care about animals, but they tend to care more about some animals, such as their own pets, than others. Regan then tries to show that reason and logic are the most important instruments for knowing what we ought to do: "one of the great challenges the ethic of care places before us is to bring our caring into line with our reason, in the sense that in time we *do* care about the pain and death of those for whom reason informs us that we *should* care" (98). Reason will tell us whom and what to care about: "reason is now empowered to demonstrate the arbitrariness of the limits imposed by an ethic of care" (97). Regan defends the view held from the time of the ancient Greeks. The emotions and the passions will lead us astray unless they are tempered by Reason.

Regan concludes "that the feminist critique of patriarchy may not be as radical as some might wish it to be" (1991, 99). Regan argues that principles of reason and logic *must* prevail over caring; and if they do, then the ethic-of-care feminist rejection of patriarchy fails because the reason/emotion dichotomy is real.

REGAN'S CONCLUSIONS

From the above we find the general conclusion that (1) an ethic-of-care feminism cannot provide an adequate ground for the rights of animals built out of several other arguments with the following conclusions: (2) ethics-of-care feminism cannot incorporate the Principle of Equality; (3) caring, the passions, or the emotions are too "chancy" a basis for ethics because they permit partiality for individual persons and may lead to injustice; (4) reason and logic offer an impartial or more objective method for telling us whom to care about; an assumption (5) reason offers a good ground for the Principle of Equality; and an auxiliary conclusion (6) the feminist ethic-of-care rejection of patriarchy fails because the reason/emotion dichotomy is real.

SOME CRITICISMS OF REGAN'S DEFENSE OF A RATIONALISTIC EPISTEMOLOGY

In the following subsections I offer a few *reasons* to think that Regan's conclusions are incorrect because his argument is invalid.

REGAN'S DEFINITION OF IMPARTIALITY IS TOO NARROW

First, we should not accept Regan's definition of impartiality as rooting the personal out of moral decision making. Impartiality actually requires that we offer sound reasons for any discrimination. Criteria concerning what constitutes morally relevant similarities and differences guide us about when it is proper to discriminate and when it is not. For example, we discriminate about punishment. We punish those who have committed a crime but not those who are innocent. We need to identify the morally relevant *situations of similarity and difference* between women and men, adults and children, human and nonhuman animals, differing cultural contexts, and so forth with the aim of showing how to consider each within a relational context.

EQUALITY CAN PERMIT SOME KINDS OF PARTIALITY

Second, recall that Regan objects to caring as a foundation for equality because people care about animals, but they tend to care more about their own pets than others. Regan carefully avoids the parallel observation that people care more about their own children than they do about other people's children. Feminists, contrary to what Regan must assume in order to claim that such partiality for one's pets is unjust, generally argue that preferences for one's own family and one's own children are not at all unjust. Thinkers such as Sara Ruddick (1989) would argue that familial preferences in caring are the very foundation of ethics.

The real question is what shall we do in case of conflict? If Regan were to take a concomitantly reasonable and caring perspective, he would see that animals have intrinsic value, have a good-of-their-own, and are "subjects-of-a-life," but that their situations differ from humans and their place in the community cannot be the same as that of our children. It simply could not be just to allow one's own child to die or suffer ill-health so that a nonhuman animal may live. To accept such a view of impartiality would be to abandon care altogether and with it, reason.

REASON CANNOT ISSUE AN "OUGHT"

Third, Regan proposes that caring is too chancy because some people care about certain people and not others and yet we say they *ought* to care. Regan claims that this "ought" has its origin in reason. Reason is supposed to be a better ground for ethics than caring because it guides caring, telling us whom we ought to care about. Yet we also know that some people are not reasonable, although we say that they *ought* to be. But reason itself cannot be used as a ground for saying one ought to be reasonable. Why then should anyone be so concerned when feminists propose an ethic of care and claim that if people do not care then they *ought* to? Just as reason cannot ground itself, care likewise cannot. Alternatively, one might propose that people should be reasonable because they ought to care about others, and people should care about others because human beings ought to be reasonable. It is reasonable to care, and caring to be reasonable. The proposition is not circular because the content of caring *and of reason* are informed by inductive experiences in the world, in the context of societies and physical environmental challenges within which human communities live. Inductive experience that makes the reason-care relationship noncircular is not "subjective" in the sense that it occurs in only one person and not others. Inductive experience must be interpersonally validated to be true.

In claiming this experiential and conceptual interrelation of caring and reason, I answer Regan's claim that the reason/emotion dichotomy is real. In my interpretation of the feminist resolution of reason/emotion, each is necessary and neither is superior in the fully developed human. Regan had claimed that what is essential to the rejection of patriarchy is the radical human-nonhuman distinction. Still, feminists need not take an all-or-nothing approach, and indeed many ethic-of-care feminists try to reject the "either/or" as it is expressed in traditional theory (Donovan 1990). We can admit that we are animals and that we share significant similarities with nonhuman animals and that these similarities are morally important. We can, however, note that there are differences between the species that situate us differently and that these differences are also morally relevant. We can look for ways to use both reason and caring in moral decision making.

REASON AND CARE CAN FUNCTION CONCOMITANTLY

Fourth, Regan (1991) claims that we must use consistency arguments in order to decide about moral rightness or wrongness. In his view this means that reason transcends care because rational consistency and appeals to logic will show the primacy of his argument that all animals are equal. But one might employ consistency arguments and still make reason and caring partners, rather than dominant and subordinate, in decision making. Consistency arguments require that we compare one moral belief to another and systematically try to adopt an ethics that does not commit us to contradictory beliefs. In any such system, some beliefs are given more weight than others. Belief in equality, universality, and impartiality is given more weight than other principles in a traditional moral system. More concrete beliefs, such as not punishing the innocent and the evil of killing, are also given greater weight than important beliefs about honesty, fidelity, and confidentiality. Feminists arguing for an ethic of care might give greater weight to beliefs about the good of giving partiality to their own children and families (which could include their pets and domestic farm animals) and still construct a consistent system. It may not be the system Regan argues for, but it could be logically consistent. The real argument is about which values are most important: a version of impartiality which grants no special status to one's own family or community or a nondiscrimination which grants partiality to some while attempting to make just decisions about the situations of others.

PERSONAL SUFFERING IS FOUNDATIONAL, ABSTRACT SUFFERING IS DERIVATIVE

Regan's arguments continue to be unnecessarily abstract and to value that abstraction. He claims that "pain and untimely death are undesirable apart from the particular identities of those who suffer or die" (1991, 97, stated twice). Yet there is no suffering and death apart from the particular people and animals who experience it. He asserts that, even though we care more about the deaths and suffering of those close to us, their suffering "would not make sense if pain and untimely death themselves were unimportant or undesirable" (97). Inductively, though, that claim appears to be false. I would mourn the suffering or death of my own child even if I did not know that anyone else ever suffered or died—a small child's grief over the death of a dear pet supports that belief. The *universal* horror at death and suffering appears to be learned from the more personal experience of it. Thus, it is universal death and suffering that would not make sense if I had not first learned to care about the death and suffering of those dear to me. He continues in the tradition of reifying pain and suffering as real things apart from those who experience it, just as "interests" come to replace the real individuals who experience well-being or not. Better that we should return to talk of the real center of moral concern: people, their families, and their communities.

Regan clearly wishes to build an alliance between feminists and animal rights advocates in *The Thee Generation* (1991). Yet he continues to argue from traditional moral theory and accepts feminism only insofar as he believes it does not challenge his own preconceptions about the way in which morality should be structured. While on the surface he appears to make some concessions to an ethic-of-care feminism and its contributions to understanding our relationship to animals, the concessions are superficial and amount to a reiteration of distrust of caring as a legitimate epistemic and ontological ground for ethics.

ECOFEMINIST VEGETARIANISM

Not all ecofeminists believe that their position requires vegetarianism. But ecofeminists share certain background beliefs about the relationship of dominant and subordinate classes and cultures, masculine and feminine stereotypes, and culture and nature that make arguments for or against ethical vegetarianism plausible. In this section, I will briefly outline the foundational beliefs that ecofeminists share, using primarily the work of Karen Warren (1990), who does not argue for ethical vegetarianism. Then, I will critically review the arguments of several ecofeminists who claim that feminists *must* be or ought to be vegetarians.

ECOFEMINIST COMMONALITIES

Ecofeminists find a psychological link between the patriarchal treatment of women and that of animals. The denial of basic rights or moral standing to women and to animals arises from similar motivations for domination. In Karen Warren's (1990) words, "what *all* ecofeminists agree about, then, is the way in which *the logic of domination* has functioned historically within patriarchy to sustain and justify the twin dominations of women and nature" (131).[10] By a "logic of domination," I interpret Warren to mean that any person or group who is motivated to dominate and subordinate others will follow a recognizable psychological pattern of expropriating power and freedom from those others and redirecting that power to the dominant's own use or to the use of the dominant class. Such action is exploitation that denies a basic good, indeed an all-important one, to the subordinate. One holding such an attitude sees the other as merely an instrument to further his or her own ends rather than regarding the other as having her or his own personal desires, ends, and intrinsic worth. Women, nature, and animals have been exploited and instrumentalized in this way in patriarchal culture. Using another for one's own ends while ignoring the being's own good fails to show proper moral respect for that being.

Warren (1987) argues for a "transformative feminism" that would broaden feminist concerns to expose "the interconnections between all systems of oppression" (18). A more complete feminism, she argues, would "provide a central theoretical place for the diversity of women's experiences, . . . acknowledge the social construction of knowledge, . . . involve rethinking what it is to be human, . . . involve recasting traditional ethical concerns to make a central place for values (for instance, care, friendship, reciprocity in relationships, appropriate trust, diversity) . . . involve challenging patriarchal bias in technology research" (18–19). Thus, a more complete feminism will incorporate concerns for nature and concerns for oppressed groups everywhere. She describes several "boundary conditions" for such a feminist ethic. Anything that furthers social domination, such as racism, sexism, classism, cannot be part of such an ethic. In her view, a properly conceived ethic is a contextualist collage that "emerges out of the very different voices of people located in different circumstances . . . [and] gives central place to the voices of women" in all their diversity (Warren 1990, 139); as such it is "inclusive." A pluralistic process, theoretical conceptions of ethics change over time. Warren makes no pretense that ethics can arise from an objective point of view, denying that such a viewpoint is possible. An adequate feminist ethic may admit talk of rights, rules, or utility in certain contexts, but would deny that morality is reducible to such talk. Finally, she calls upon feminist ethicists to reconceive the nature of our humanity and to reject "as either meaningless or currently untenable any gender-free or gender-neutral description of humans, ethics, and ethical decision making" (141). Humans fundamentally are in relation to each other and to their natural environment. She identifies the foregoing as the primary constituents of an ecofeminist ethic.

CAROL ADAMS' AFFIRMATION OF ANIMAL RIGHTS AND ETHICAL VEGANISM

Although Karen Warren does not argue for ethical vegetarianism as necessary to an adequate ecofeminist ethic, Carol Adams sees the connection as essential. For twenty-five years, Carol Adams has argued that feminists should be vegetarians (for example, 1975, 1976, 1990, 1991, 1993); she is herself a practicing vegan. Among her writings, "The Feminist Traffic in Animals" (1993) most vividly illustrates the alliance she has formed with the animal rights movement. She has also appeared with Tom Regan and other animal rights advocates in conferences on the topic.[11]

In this section I review Adams' work and show that her view is entirely traditionalist in its orientation while only the rhetoric she employs is feminist. She assumes that no inconsistencies exist between a feminist defense of the moral standing of animals and a moral rights defense. So, she adopts a rights defense and its implications. Yet, she chooses feminist rhetoric where it seems to fit in with a traditional moral rights view. Then she claims her view is, in essence, feminist.

In her 1993 article, Adams specifically argues that feminists must accept animal rights and become ethical vegans. Adams uses many of the important terms of feminist rhetoric to build her analogy between the situations of food animals and the situations of women. Thinking about women as *naturally* given to any particular role objectifies them as the "other," and thinking about animals as naturally consumable likewise objectifies them. Yet "nothing inherent in a cow's existence . . . necessitates her future fate as hamburger . . ." (202). Women have been a subordinated social group, and animals are, too. That subordination has arisen in "the process of 'naturalizing' the political" (203). She argues that "'human' de facto represents white (human) maleness and 'other' represents that which white human maleness negates: other races, sexes, or species" (Adams, 1993, 203). The claim is that to reject white male patriarchy one must reject the self-other dichotomy. Adams also reiterates the feminist dogma that "the personal is political" (196) and believes that the attempt to see animals as different is to classify them as "other" and in so doing to privatize or depoliticize the eating of animals.

Adams (1991) makes this specific regarding animals, women, and domination (126–29). Through analysis of literary texts, Adams demonstrates a Western cultural link between meat eating and strength by showing a mythical association of masculinity with bellicosity and the supposed "need" men have to eat meat (Adams 1990). In contrast, vegetable eating has been associated with femininity and weakness (Adams 1990). In all her work thus far, Adams begins from the assumption that animals are of moral concern and presents no systematic defense for the position that feminists are morally required to espouse vegetarianism or work for a vegetarian world, believing that "by exposing the way violence worked, a feminist ethics is already in place to respond to such violence" (Adams 1993, personal communication). She claims that these cultural and psychological links make vegetarianism morally necessary to both feminism and ecofeminism.

Her analogy must surely give any feminist pause to wonder whether she has a point. But even a traditional, "common sense," anti-cruelty view can outlaw the kind of inhumane treatment that animals receive in intensive agricultural systems today. Adams seems to take the stronger view that any meat eating in a society where vegan lifestyles are possible would be wrong, even if the animals were humanely raised and painlessly killed after having enjoyed a good life. Although it is not clear whether *she* believes her feminist view of "animal rights" is founded on or is at least consistent with traditional moral rights theory, I think it cannot be otherwise. As a test, could her "rights" position rely on some other contextual or ethic-of-care ground? It is difficult to see that it can. The reasons she gives for condemning meat eating are more consistent with a neo-Kantian moral rights theory *ala* Regan than those given by ethic-of-care feminists such as Josephine Donovan (1990) discussed above.

Second, several aspects of her writings make Adams' view systematically most consistent with Regan's. She affirms the universality of ethical veganism, equality as sameness, and an absolutism in that ethical veganism appears virtually exceptionless as a moral imperative. In all of these aspects, she echoes traditional moral theory. She equates human autonomy and animal liberty and sees no significant differences between conditions that oppress humans and those that oppress animals. In this, she apparently agrees with Regan about the superseding value of abstract interests in not suffering pain over the value of the pain of those in close personal relationships with us. Echoing Kant's (1785) practical imperative to "Treat persons always as ends-in-themselves and never as a means only," she condemns *using* animals to satisfy our needs: "without our needing them . . . they would not exist" (Adams 1993, 203). Likewise, Adams embraces a strict abolitionism concerning the consumption of animals. At least in her rhetoric, her absolutism is most consistent with a Kantian assertion of perfect duties derived from categorical imperatives. Presumably eating one slice of bologna a year would be just as immoral as eating a quarter-pounder three times a day every day for a year.[12]

Very often the reasons she gives depart from those most often associated with feminist ethics: Feminists most often reject dichotomies, but she sees justice and charity in opposition to one another (Adams 1993, 205). Whereas feminists commonly argue for overcoming dualisms, she embraces the dualistic ontology of self and other. She claims that feminists who object to imposing ethical vegetarianism on others "are naïve thinkers. . . . They wrongly conclude that there is such a thing as neutrality" (1993, 214). "No objective stance exists from which to survey the traffic in animals. Either we eat them or we do not" (1993, 198). In claiming there is no neutral ground, Adams embraces the "either/or" of the kind of absolutist ethics that she herself wishes to reject when she uses feminist rhetoric.

Adams (1993) argues for universality and moral objectivism and against the cultural relativism in the traditional way: she claims relativism is an invidious foundation of the pluralism adopted by many feminists. The pluralistic feminist sees "a universal vegetarianism . . . as a white woman's imposing her 'dietary' concerns on women of color" (211). The pluralist claims that respect for other cultures requires respect for their values, and food practices constitute an important reflection of those values. Adams rejoins that "we do not embrace nondominant cultural traditions that, for instance, oppress women" (211), and thereby illustrates her equation of human liberty and autonomy with animal liberty and advocates a cross-cultural objectivism.

For the moment, I leave aside the question of whether Adams' claims are well-founded. All I wish to show here is that her arguments are most consistent when seen as arising from a traditional moral rights theoretic. That being so, Adams' arguments rely on the truth of traditional rights arguments for ethical vegetarianism. Because these traditional rights arguments fail, as I show in the next chapter, her claims concerning the imperative to ethical veganism also fail.

OTHER ECOFEMINIST VEGETARIANS

Lori Gruen (1993) claims there is a "practical connection between the liberation of women and that of animals" (82). Some feminists claim that respect for the diversity of cultural traditions requires a nonjudgmental attitude about food. But in her view the reasons offered in support of serving meat and other animal products at feminist gatherings are "rationalizations [that] ignore the infringement of an animal's 'right' to live a pain-free life and fail to recognize that cultural traditions are exactly those institutions at which legitimate feminist critiques are aimed" (82). Gruen uses scare quotes around the word 'right' to indicate that she uses the word operationally, rather than to indicate any overarching appeal to traditional theory. In her view, "ecofeminist practice is a revolt against control, power, production, and competition in all of their manifestations" (84). A shift in values is needed to encompass a "methodological humility" that she describes as "a method of deep respect for difference" that requires us to "operate under the assumption that there may be something happening that cannot be immediately understood" (84). Gruen seems to be claiming that methodological humility will help us to see the connections between the oppression of women and that of animals and thereby ground the rejection of meat eating.

On the other hand, isn't it possible that something else may be happening among women and animals in other cultures that we do not immediately understand? If one believes that all reasons one might offer in support of certain food traditions are mere excuses, then the method of understanding cannot even begin. Perhaps it is *our tradition* rather than theirs that makes us see the relation of food, animals, and humans as inescapably oppressive.

Marti Kheel (1985), founder of Feminists for Animal Rights, takes a pragmatic approach to the moral tradition. Although she argues from an ecological feminist perspective, she perceives appeals to rights arguments as "a necessary tactical device within our current society" (147). Her main concern is to bring the ethical emotions and feelings into the fray. She argues against a hierarchy that pits reason against emotion in rights theory and in newer holistic views of environmental ethics. She sees the efforts to defeat the old hierarchies as simply producing new ones: Whereas traditionally only humans had inherent value, animal rights advocates claim that nonhumans and humans also have inherent value, but the rest of nature does not. Traditionally, nature does not have inherent value because the ground of value must be sentience, which enables us to understand the interests of the being. Thus, the environment can have no value of its own, but is valued only as an instrument for sentient beings—a new hierarchy is born.

Environmentalists object to the claim that nature has no inherent value. Instead, we must look upon all life *holistically* with the realization that rivers, streams, mountains, and forests belong to the web of life as they function in ecosystems. As such, their value cannot be abstracted from that of the living being. Kheel notes that both holism and rights reject feelings, emotions, and inclinations. She argues for their restoration to moral epistemology because feelings and emotions are characteristic of individuals and so exist in the whole as well. Kheel proposes as an alternative "a concept of holism that perceives nature . . . as comprising individual beings that are part of a *dynamic* web of interconnections in which feelings, emotions, and inclinations . . . play an integral role" (140–41).

On the question of the ground for animal rights, Kheel notes that Regan's appeal to "marginal cases" relies not on reason, but on intuition or feeling. She argues that "we cannot even begin to talk about the issue of ethics unless we admit that we care (or feel something)" (144). Following Robin Morgan (1982), Kheel claims that we must ground ethics on a "unified sensibility" that blends feeling and reason as it arises from personal experience. Thus, in trying to decide about ethical vegetarianism we might visit a factory farm or a slaughterhouse to see if we still *feel* the same way about meat eating: "When we are physically removed from the direct impact of our moral decisions—that is, when we cannot see, smell, or hear their results—we deprive ourselves of sensory stimuli which may be important in guiding us in our ethical choices. If we, ourselves, do not want to witness, let alone participate in, the slaughter of the animals we eat, we ought, perhaps, to question the morality of indirectly paying someone else to do this on our behalf "(145). She encourages us to make our choices a "circular affair" by seeking to understand from personal experience. These experiences should evoke feelings that may cause us to re-evaluate our *thinking*. We should, in this way, be more capable of becoming involved "in the *whole* process of our moral decisions" (145). I interpret Kheel to mean that thinking, feeling, and experience should be unified in the judgment process, but that a dialectic among them will go on to make changes in our beliefs about the rightness or wrongness of certain actions, choices, or practices.

Kheel's moral epistemology extends beyond adding feeling and emotion as icing on the cake. Her emphasis and that of other feminists on the importance of care at times appears to tip the balance away from reason. From a practical point-of-view, though, talking up care and feeling has to be done because there is so much distrust of the emotions in moral philosophy. Kheel clearly appeals for balance and a "down-to-earth" experiential ground for valuation.

Unfortunately, it isn't clear how personal experience at the slaughterhouse could move us to the conclusion that we should give up meat. Most slaughterhouse workers remain omnivores. We might simply say that we should work for more humane conditions, and in fact Temple Grandin (1989a,b) has made it her life's work to create humane slaughterhouses in which cattle and other animals can be painlessly killed without any foreknowledge of their death. Supposing we ourselves *are* willing to kill a chicken—a relatively common experience for women living in rural areas. Unlike slaughterhouse workers, these women cannot be dismissed as callused by their work. Kheel might conceivably say that the rural woman does *no* wrong given her personal experience, feeling, reason and context, whereas slaughterhouse workers and urban dwellers do wrong to animals because these workers are either physically or psychologically cut off from their feelings. Somehow I doubt that she *would* say this, but there might be some reason to think the contrast points up an important moral difference. We do not think it is *as wrong* to kill only what we need for ourselves (Kheel does praise animals for this), as it is to kill for a living or to kill for others. Or, put another way, it appears to be *better*, or somehow more virtuous, for each of us to kill only what we need to eat. But, why should this be so?

First of all, such a belief could reflect an affirmation of our similarity to animals, who also kill only what they need. In killing only the meat we *need* to eat, we affirm our equality with animals. Of course, if we need no meat and agricultural cultivation does not damage the habitat of other animals and plants, then we should kill only plants and not more than we need of them, too. This belief about satiety and economy also has ancient roots in virtue ethics. The vices of gluttony and waste are condemned in Christianity and other world religions as well. Abstinence from food—fasting—is regarded as virtuous and saintly in the history of the Christian church and in many other religious traditions.

Kheel's view expresses an ecofeminist holism that cannot be reduced to rights or utilitarianism. I have illustrated ways in which her view also bears some affinities with a virtue ethic. She asks individuals to place themselves in situations where they can learn to feel and to think about their choices, presuming the experiences will result in moral improvement. Although she does not identify virtues and vices, she might well agree that her view does uphold virtues of economy and condemn the vices of gluttony and waste.

DEANE CURTIN'S CONTEXTUAL MORAL VEGETARIANISM

Deane Curtin (1991) has also argued that ecofeminist insights about the treatment of nonhuman animals and the environment cannot be adequately expressed in the language of rights. He develops his own view on ecofeminist vegetarianism that most closely resembles a virtue ethics in its emphasis on looking at who a person is rather than what she does.

The affirmation of animal rights by ecofeminists commits them to a framework that excludes the central tenets of ecofeminism. Tom Regan's argument in *The Thee Generation* (1991) that care cannot be an adequate ground for animal rights validates one point in Curtin's counterargument: rights theory requires the ascendancy of reason over emotion, but feminism generally rejects that division. Curtin claims that attempts to ground ethical vegetarianism in animal rights "are better understood conceptually in terms of an ethic of care" (1991, 65). Curtin then develops his own contextual view of moral vegetarianism as a commitment to defining oneself in relation to the food eaten and to limiting violence. His advocacy of vegetarianism is contextual because "there may be some contexts in which another response is appropriate. Though I am committed to moral vegetarianism, I cannot say that I would never kill an animal for food. Would I not kill an animal to provide food for my son if he were starving? Would I not generally prefer the death of a bear to the death of a loved one? I am sure I would. The point of a contextualist ethic is that one need not treat all interests equally as if one had no relationship to any of the parties" (1991, 69–70).

Curtin's view is striking and appealing in its reference to the development of *healthy personhood* as the goal of a good life. He argues that the self is discovered in the ordinary experiences of food in daily life. The focus on the ordinary blurs the distinction between the moral and the aesthetic and creates a union of the mind and body through choosing, eating, and experiencing food. Rather than envisioning oneself as an autonomous agent who lives over against the world, fending off domination by others, the healthy self has "the power to direct one's life [through] accepting herself as body" (1992a, 8). Paying attention to our own personal experiences as we grow, prepare, and eat food enables us to become self-aware and to develop as healthy persons. "We are," he reminds us, "what we eat in a most literal, bodily way. Our bodies literally are food transformed into flesh, tendon, blood, and bone" (11). We distinguish food from the merely edible. "The classification of something as food means it is understood as something made to become part of who we are. Classifying an edible as food means we have foreknowledge that it will become us bodily. . . . Food stands in a special relationship to the self" (9). He contrasts the objectified discontinuity of food practice in the modern United States with a "participatory" and relational view that sees food as defining the self. In objectifying food as something other than ourselves, we affirm disconnection with the world, its temporality, its transience, and its ordinariness. Yet the real self lives in time and in a flux of moments that come and return in the ordinariness of daily meals (1992a,b).

Curtin (1992a,b) adds another dimension by linking vegetarianism to the development of a *healthy self:* the affirmation of nonviolence as a "moral direction" to be consciously chosen. This moral direction he grounds in a politicized ethic of care (1991) and later connects it to Buddhist conceptions of the food-self relation (1991, 1992a,b). Nel Noddings (1984) argues that mutual responsiveness is required for a moral relationship to occur. Curtin disagrees. Such a view excessively privatizes the experiences of women. The ethic of care, he claims, must be politicized to permit a generalized caring about even those who cannot return our care or reciprocate in any way. Otherwise, care cannot ground an adequate environmental ethic. Since mountains, rivers, and streams cannot respond to our needs, a caring ethic that *requires* reciprocity in the relationship will also fall short of permitting us to care about distant people and animals.

Curtin connects caring with the commitment to reducing violence in one's life. He acknowledges that violence cannot be eliminated, for we must kill plants to eat and many of our ordinary actions result in killing unseen organisms and other living things. And, "a contextualist ethic should not give in to the illusion that there is a universalizable program of caring that will magically alleviate all suffering" (1992b, 135). Whether or not one *ought* morally to choose vegetarianism depends on context, that is, the society in which we live: "As a 'contextual moral vegetarian,' I cannot refer to an absolute moral rule that prohibits meat eating under all circumstances" (1991, 69). Thus, Curtin expresses reasons to embrace vegetarianism that affirm most, if not all, of the ways feminists wish to approach ethics. He affirms the integration of care and reason, finds meaning in daily life and ordinariness that integrates body and spirit, and rejects dichotomies, universality, and absolutism as well as rule-bound ethics. He proposes nonviolence and nondomination as "moral directions" for healthy selfhood, and these attitudes closely resemble traits of character commonly called virtues.[13]

Curtin has argued that moral vegetarianism "is completely compelling as an expression of an ecological ethic of care . . . for economically well-off persons in technologically advanced countries" (1991, 70). Because Curtin's view is the best developed feminist account of ethical vegetarianism and I argue that feminists cannot consistently adopt an ethical vegetarianism, I return to his work in chapter 7. Although Curtin rejects most formal aspects of the moral tradition, he praises certain attitudes and virtues that bridge the tradition. I shall argue that ethical vegetarianism is nevertheless inconsistent with his fuller affirmation of feminism.

In the following chapter, I show how traditional moral arguments, in particular, but all arguments for ethical vegetarianism in general, presuppose the equality of animals and humans and nondiscrimination based on species, gender, age, class, race, or physical ability. Further, I show how moral arguments for ethical vegetarianism that are extended from traditional moral theory become self-contradictory because these arguments precipitate discrimination among these groups.

CHAPTER 4

A FEMINIST ARGUMENT AGAINST ETHICAL VEGETARIANISM

HOW TRADITIONAL MORAL THEORY FAILS

Singer, Regan, and virtually all other philosophers defending the moral status of animals claim that animals are our equals and that we may not kill them for food. According to Peter Singer (1975), we may not use their products unless we could be sure that these products are obtained under painless conditions. Singer's utilitarian position would permit some people to eat animals or their products if they have a strong welfare-interest (say, for reasons of ill health), but these would be exceptional cases, on grounds that are apparently the same as offered by Tom Regan (1983).[1] Regan's rights position allows certain people to consume meat as exceptional cases based on what he dubs the Liberty Principle:

> Provided that all those involved are treated with respect, and assuming that no special considerations obtain, any innocent individual has the right to act to avoid being made worse-off even if doing so harms other innocents (1983, 333).

Being made to starve or suffer a significant decline in health and vigor would make us worse-off, and Regan accedes that if some humans have a strong welfare-interest in consuming meat or animal products, this would excuse them from a duty to be vegetarians. But Regan clearly thinks most people do not fall into such a category. He briefly discusses protein complementation and then dismisses the argument from nutrition: "Certain amino acids are essential for our health. Meat isn't. We cannot, therefore, defend meat eating on the grounds that we will ruin our health if we don't eat it or even that we will run a very serious risk of doing so if we abstain" (1983, 337).

The question is, to whom does that "we" refer? Traditional morality claims to prescribe for everyone—not merely for some; its rules are supposed to be universal. Because its rules are universal and rights-holders are equal, the rules should also be impartial. All mature and rational persons regardless of their age, sex, race, and other irrelevant factors are supposed to be able to follow a universal rule—or at least to be capable of being taught to do so. Traditional moral theories assume the moral equality and the general interchangeability of persons regardless of age, sex, race, and so forth. Ethical vegetarians and ethical vegans suppose that all of us could adopt such diets if we choose.

In making these assumptions, ethical vegetarians posit a moral norm that should be consistent with physiological norms. "Moral norms" are rules and standards meant to guide the conduct of beings who have the capacity for morality. Moral norms and physiological norms should not be confused, even though both imply significant value claims. A "physiological norm," as it is intended here, picks out some fact or material aspect about the world, such as, "it is the norm for males to produce more testosterone than estrogen." We might pick out many more traits that are common for the human species. Abnormal physiology need not and should not be taken to mean moral inferiority or even illness, although it will sometimes impair function. People born with webbed fingers or toes, extra fingers or even no fingers at all are neither morally inferior nor ill, although their physical function differs from that usually seen. Nondiscrimination requires that, insofar as possible, society should eliminate moral, social, or legal constraints that will cause extraordinary persons to suffer an increased burden in their attempts to function in society. We provide ramps for those who use wheelchairs, for instance. Nondiscrimination is the attempt by fair-minded people to affirm the equal worth of each member of the moral community. No single group can simply assume that its own practices are the only right ones, or even the best ones. Nondiscrimination also requires that moral norms distribute burdens and benefits equitably among groups. It is wrong, for example, to set out greater punishments for offenders of one race than for another. If the moral norm or rule prescribing vegetarian or vegan diets is truly nondiscriminatory, it should not require greater or very much greater burdens for some groups because of aspects about themselves that cannot be changed and that are thought to be neutral to the interests served by the rule.[2]

The moral rule requiring vegetarianism is quite otherwise. It does systematically impose greater burdens on some. Although most men age 20–50 in industrialized countries can choose to be vegetarians without significant risk or burdens, the same cannot be said for other people identifiable by characteristics over which they have no choice or control: infants, children, adolescents, gestating and lactating women, and some elderly people. Inextricably bound up with this male physiological norm is a presupposed cultural norm that is biased against many people living in ethnic, cultural, economic, and environmental circumstances unlike those in which a vegan ideal can be successfully realized. That cultural norm also presupposes a society largely structured on wealth generated from unsustainable environmental, agricultural, and industrial practices.

In what follows, I explain why arguments for a stringent ethical vegetarianism must suppose that all or almost all ethical vegans and vegetarians have bodies approximating that of an adult male between the ages of twenty and fifty. This is the "male physiological norm" and it is biased against females, children, and the elderly. Later in this chapter in "The Cultural Norm of Wealth," I discuss the similarly biased class, cultural, and genetic norms that are concomitantly bound up with this male physiological norm. But from a nutritional point-of-view, what we should eat to maintain health and well-being depends to a great extent on where we live and to some degree on our genetic inheritance.

Ethical vegans and vegetarians often bypass concerns about such biases with the rejoinder that women and children can easily supplement their vegetarian diets (see for instance, Adams 1995; Donovan 1995; Gaard and Gruen 1995; Pluhar 1992; Varner 1994a). Processed, fortified foods and supplement tablets are widely available. Research also shows that vegetarian diets have health benefits. In "Counterbalancing Considerations," I show why these rejoinders remain biased in assuming a male ideal body and a cultural norm of wealth.

Arguments extended from traditional moral theory rely on a supposed "average human being" quite capable of switching to a vegan or vegetarian diet with the proper will, but he turns out to look very healthy, wealthy, Western, and well-fed. Women, children, and others are dealt with by granting them "special dispensations" from the usual moral rules that would obtain in the ethical vegan's ideal world. Therefore, the final two sections of this chapter show how such a structure of ethical thinking about food, nutrition, and health plays into the logic of domination and reinforces the unacceptability of the female body and participates in opening up feminine responses such as anorexia nervosa and bulimia.

THE MALE PHYSIOLOGICAL NORM

That nutritional needs differ with stages of life and between the sexes is well-documented in the medical and nutrition literature. "Semivegetarian diets usually pose little or no nutritional risk. Dietary nutrient intakes are likely to be adequate" (Dwyer 1993b, 175). Vegan diets, on the other hand, present greater dietary risk than lactoovovegetarian diets, even though these also pose risks for some groups. Looking at differences in risk among these groups illuminates differences in physiology between women and men and between adults, children, and the old. Then, the biased perspective of the traditional arguments for ethical vegetarianism should become clearer.

DIFFERENCES IN NUTRITIONAL REQUIREMENTS AMONG HUMANS

The "First International Congress on Vegetarian Nutrition" was held in Washington, D.C., on March 16–18, 1987, and the "Second International Congress" was held in Arlington, Virginia, on June 28–July 1, 1992. Proceedings for these conferences were published in single issues of the *American Journal of Clinical Nutrition* (1988: 48:3 and 1994:59[supp.]). In the last several years, many comprehensive reviews have also appeared in the literature on the risks and benefits of vegan and vegetarian diets (for example, Dwyer 1988, 1991; Dwyer and Loew 1994; Havala and Dwyer 1988, 1993; University of California 1993). Dwyer (1988) specifically addresses the health benefits of vegetarianism. A number of reviews of health problems associated with nutrition in women, children, the elderly, and "minorities" have also been published. For example, a 1991 supplement to the *American Journal of Clinical Nutrition* was devoted to a series of papers and reviews on the calcium requirement by prominent researchers in the field. A primary concern with the calcium requirement for women is its relation to osteoporosis (Dawson-Hughes 1991; Pollitzer and Anderson 1989; Peacock 1991; Rodysill 1987). Reviews have also appeared in several journals on the recent research in the role of iron in childhood development, in pregnancy and lactation (Bothwell *et al.* 1989; Dallman 1989; Hercberg and Galan 1989, 1992; McDonald and Keen 1988; Parks and Wharton 1989). Pediatric nutrition is thoroughly covered in Suskind and Lewinter-Suskind (1993) and in Queen and Lang (1993). Munro *et al.* (1987) review the nutritional requirements of the elderly. Review of the literature on vitamin B_{12} deficiency and on the availability of B_{12} from supplements appear in Doyle *et al.* (1989); Herbert (1984, 1988); and Herbert and Subak-Sharpe (1990). Extensive reviews of studies on all of the known vitamin and mineral requirements appear in the *Recommended Daily Allowances* (National Research Council 1989b). Nutritional vulnerabilities of gestating and lactating women are thoroughly discussed in the reports of the Institute of Medicine (1990, 1991). Genetic differences that concern diet and health are discussed by the National Research Council (1989a). In December 1992, the National Academy of Sciences, Institute of Medicine, held a symposium on "Nutrition and Minority Health: The Interplay of Food, Culture, Genetics, and Environment" and their findings were reported in Patlak (1993). These reviews, in general, refer to findings from settings in industrialized societies where foods are fortified and available in abundance.

Scrimshaw (1991) reports on iron deficiency in areas of the world where the variety and supply of food is limited. Soysa (1987) has reviewed the nutritional status of women in nonindustrialized nations, and comments about the nutritional status of women in other cultures may also be found in Pollitzer and Anderson (1989) and Wardlaw and Insel (1993). A summary of the findings from these and other studies follows; all of the reviews and studies cited illustrate the well-established physiological differences among various groups by age, sex, race, ethnicity, and cultural circumstance. In addition, these reviews give us insight into the "vegan ideal" as an adult male who lives in a high-tech society and is very likely white and middle or upper class.

In the following few pages, I summarize first the differences in vitamin and mineral requirements that are established for stage of life; that is, for children and adolescents versus adults, pregnant and lactating women versus adult males, and elderly persons versus people aged 20–50. Then, because our dietary choices can create situations that require more attention to vitamin and mineral needs in these age groups, I go on to discuss the particular vulnerabilities of each dietary group (vegan or lactoovovegetarian) to certain nutritional deficits.

NUTRITIONAL VULNERABILITIES BY STAGE OF LIFE

Infants and young children have higher energy, vitamin, and mineral needs than adults do because they are continuously growing and adding new tissue to their bodies. They also have smaller stomachs than adults and need more efficient delivery of calories in relatively concentrated form. Adolescents also need diets that are dense in nutrients per kilocalorie because they undergo the pubertal growth spurt. The onset of menstruation in females increases their iron needs, and the need for protein increases because the body size is increasing rapidly (Dwyer 1993a). Because bone mass is being accumulated, calcium needs remain higher until about age twenty-five. The RDAs for adolescents are "considerably higher for adolescents than they are for younger children or adults, especially if they are expressed on a nutrients-per-calorie basis" (Dwyer 1993a, 257). "Sex differences in nutrient needs become especially pronounced during adolescence" (258). Pregnant adult women have greater protein, calcium, iron, vitamin C, vitamin D, vitamin E, thiamin, riboflavin, niacin, vitamin B_6, folate, vitamin B_{12}, phosphorus, magnesium, zinc, selenium, and iodide needs than adult males, and breastfeeding women have requirements that are higher still for almost all of these nutrients (National Research Council 1989b). Pregnant or lactating adolescents have requirements beyond those of older women because their own bodies are still growing and peak bone mass has not been reached.

In the United States, some adolescents are at higher risk for nutritional problems than others. "They are largely poor, rural, and/or minority groups, especially African Americans, Hispanics, and Native Americans" (Dwyer 1993a, 260). Adolescents with chronic degenerative diseases, "emotional problems that precipitate eating disorders, mental retardation, mental illness, and alcohol or drug abuse" also are at risk for poor nutritional status (Dwyer 1993a, 260).

Persons over age fifty have different requirements for several nutrients as reflected in the RDAs (National Research Council 1989b; Munro *et al.* 1987).

NUTRITIONAL VULNERABILITIES FOR VEGANS

Virtually all nutritional authorities agree that young children may be at greater risk for health problems on vegan diets than are adult males (Calkins 1988; Jacobs and Dwyer 1988; Dagnelie *et al.* 1989; Havala and Dwyer 1988, 1993; Truesdell and Acosta 1985; Dwyer 1993b; *Journal of the American Medical Association* 1974; Dwyer *et al.* 1978, 1980; Wardlaw and Insel 1993; Shull *et al.* 1977; Dwyer 1991; Dwyer and Loew 1994). As Johanna T. Dwyer of Tufts University Schools of Medicine and Nutrition writes: "Vegetarianism in children deserves special attention because diets that sustain adults in good health are not necessarily appropriate for infants, young children, or adolescents" (1993b, 171).[3] Phyllis B. Acosta, of Florida State University's Department of Nutrition and Food Science, states concerns in stronger terms: "Eating practices that promote health in the adult may have detrimental effects on growth and health status of the infant and young child" (1988, 872). Dwyer's (1991) comprehensive review of 135 sources details specific concerns for infants, children, women, and the elderly in the United States and Europe. Vegan infants and toddlers "may fail to thrive because their diets are too low in energy and too high in bulk" (Dwyer 1991, 76). Vegan diets are high in fibrous foods that have high volume but are low in calories. A toddler's stomach may simply be too small to contain enough of these foods to provide sufficient calories for growth (Dwyer 1991, 1993b; Truesdell and Acosta 1985). The prestigious vegetarian cookbook, *The New Laurel's Kitchen,* does not recommend vegan diets for infants and children (Robertson *et al.* 1986, 416–417). Parents of vegan children must take extra care to see that their children get sufficient quantities of vitamins D and B_{12}, iron, calcium, and zinc (Dwyer 1991, 1993b; Jacobs and Dwyer 1988).

Breastfed infants from age 0–6 months are vegans. Human milk is high in calcium, low in iron and zinc, and has levels of vitamins D and B_{12} (and other nutrients) that depend on the mother's level. In most places in the world, breastfeeding has many advantages for infants and mothers. Studies report that breast-fed infants have fewer gastrointestinal, respiratory, and ear infections (Institute of Medicine 1991, 166–67). "Breast-feeding appears to be protective against food allergies" and is associated with lower incidence of some types of skin rashes in infants (Institute of Medicine 1991, 167–68).[4] Death rates for breast-fed infants are much lower, "such that the postneonatal death rates of breast-fed infants continued to remain at least half those of bottle-fed infants" for the period 1850 to 1950 (Institute of Medicine 1991, 172).

Vegans who are breast-feeding their infants may have reduced levels of vitamin D and B_{12} in their own bodies and in their milk. Supplementation for these nutrients is recommended not only to protect the woman's health but to reduce risk to the nursing infant (Dwyer 1991, 75–76; see also Institute of Medicine 1991, 13, 140, 232). In pregnant women, "certain dietary practices that restrict or prohibit the consumption of an important source of nutrients, such as avoidance of all animal foods or of vitamin D–fortified milk, increase the risk of inadequate nutrient intake" (Institute of Medicine 1990, 18). Pregnant vegan women may be at greater nutritional risk for "inadequate weight gain, low protein intake, inadequate iron intake with resulting anemias, low calcium, zinc, and vitamin B_{12} intakes, and in some instances low vitamin D, zinc and iodide intakes" (Dwyer 1991, 75–76). Because the health of a fetus depends upon the health of the individual woman carrying it, these factors may pose a fetal risk as well.

Elderly people also have different requirements for several nutrients (Munro *et al.* 1987). Chronic degenerative diseases are more common. Risks of heart disease and hypertension are decreased among those who have followed a vegan or vegetarian lifestyle for a long period of time; however, risks for other chronic diseases such as osteoporosis and deficiencies for vitamin B_{12}, D, and other nutrient deficiencies secondary to atrophic gastritis may be increased (Dwyer and Loew 1994).

Notwithstanding these risks, Dwyer (1991) and Dwyer and Loew (1994) maintain that all risks for vegans in the United States can be overcome with a well-planned and well-supplemented diet. What does "well-planned" mean? Here I quote more fully the context of Dwyer's (1991) statement:

> For those who wish to progress to a vegan diet that includes no ani-mal foods whatsoever, additional care in dietary planning is needed. In addition to iron and zinc, unplanned vegan diets are often low in kilocalories, calcium, and are always low in vitamin B_{12} and vitamin D unless supplementary sources of these vitamins are provided, since plant foods contain no known sources of these vitamins. The assistance of a registered dietitian is helpful, since a good deal of skill in planning and familiarity with unconventional food sources is needed by omnivores who wish to alter their dietary intakes in this way. Certainly, if the individual in question is an infant, child, preg-nant or lactating woman, over sixty-five years of age, recovering from an illness, or a chronic sufferer of a disease, dietetic consulta-tion is highly advisable in order to incorporate these additional con-siderations into dietary planning and to avoid or circumvent adverse nutritional consequences. Several good articles are available to guide counseling efforts for vulnerable groups . . . (82–83).

Dwyer writes three more pages about specific requirements and concerns, which supplement the outline of risks and benefits earlier in the paper.

Vitamin B_{12}. All vegans must supplement their diet with a source of vitamin B_{12} that is bioavailable, that is, in a form the body can use, because this essential vitamin is not found in any plant food: "There is no active vitamin B_{12} in any-thing that grows out of the ground" (Herbert 1988, 852). Herbert (1984, 1988) recounts as well the serious consequences of not supplementing a vegan diet: "Careful studies from England . . . on several hundred vegans showed that they all eventually get vitamin B_{12} deficiency disease with anemia and pancy-topenia, low white counts, low red counts, low platelet counts, and slowed DNA synthesis" (1988, 857). Although vitamin B_{12} is manufactured in the human colon, it is not absorbable there, so vegans must obtain the vitamin from their diet.[5] Supplement sources are not always reliable. In 1988, Herbert reported that assays from his laboratory of common supplements sold in stores contain useless analogs, many of which actually block true vitamin B_{12} uptake.

Herbert (1984) explains why many women are more vulnerable to B_{12} deficiencies than men: "During the latter half of pregnancy, the fetus removes approximately 0.2 µg of vitamin B_{12} daily from maternal stores" (352). Lactat-ing women lose 0.45 µg to 0.56 µg of vitamin B_{12} per day (National Research

Council 1989b, 163). So, the RDA is twenty percent higher for pregnant women and thirty percent higher for lactating women, whether or not they are vegetarians, than for other adults. For vegan women, adequate B_{12} concentration in breast milk depends on adequate supplementation. Specker *et al.* (1990) found that vitamin B_{12} concentrations were lower in the milk of vegan women who avoided supplements, and the longer the women had been on vegan diets (median time was seventy-two months), the lower the vitamin B_{12} concentrations were in their milk. Lower concentrations were, in turn, correlated with biochemical signs of vitamin B_{12} deficiency in their infants.

Because of widespread multivitamin and mineral supplementation, vitamin B_{12} deficiency is rare in industrialized countries. When it occurs in childhood, it is "usually due to nutritional deficiency rather than to congenital metabolic disease" (Davis *et al.* 1981). But, in the last twenty-five years, alternative life-styles and vegan diets have become more popular (Davis *et al.* 1981; Dagnelie *et al.* 1989). Accompanying this trend is an increasing number of reports of vitamin B_{12} deficiencies in breast-fed infants of vegan mothers living in the United States, Europe, Australia, and other parts of the industrialized world (Lampkin *et al.* 1966; Srikantia and Reddy 1967; Lampkin and Saunders 1969; Williams and Ireland 1977; Frader *et al.* 1978; Higginbottom et al. 1978; Anonymous 1979; Rendle-Short *et al.* 1979; Wighton *et al.* 1979; Davis *et al.* 1981; Lacroix *et al.* 1981; Hoey *et al.* 1982; Johnson and Roloff 1982; Sadowitz *et al.* 1986; Sklar 1986; Silberstein *et al.* 1987; Stollhoff and Schulte 1987; Dagnelie *et al.* 1989; Doyle *et al.* 1989; Specker *et al.* 1990; Kuhne *et al.* 1991; Michaud *et al.* 1992; Monfort-Gouraud *et al.* 1993). Dwyer (1991) and Doyle *et al.* (1989) cite several additional case studies of infants and mothers with vitamin B_{12} dietary deficiency.

Lactovegetarians or lactoovovegetarians are not, in general, at great risk of vitamin B_{12} deficiency because they can obtain enough vitamin B_{12} from eggs, milk or cheese (Dwyer and Loew 1994).[6] On the other hand, vegans living in developing countries may also be at lower risk for vitamin B_{12} deficiency because their vegetables cannot be washed thoroughly enough to remove the bacterial contamination that generates vitamin B_{12} (Dwyer 1991).

With aging, atrophic gastritis increases and diminishes absorption of vitamin B_{12}, iron, calcium and other nutrients (Herbert and Subak-Sharpe 1990; Dwyer and Loew 1994). Lowik *et al.* (1990) studied forty-four apparently healthy Dutch vegetarians, aged 65–97 years, who refrained from all meat, fish, and poultry, and found that the men in particular had "aged successfully with respect to cardiovascular risk factors," but that these vegetarians had marginal levels of iron, zinc, and vitamin B_{12} (600). Dietary treatment of vitamin B_{12}

deficiency may not be successful in the elderly, and reversal often requires injection of the vitamin to circumvent the problem of gastric malabsorption (National Research Council 1989b; Herbert and Subak-Sharpe 1990).

Vitamin D. Vegans do not drink milk or eat dairy products. In Western countries this means the loss of a significant supplemented source of vitamin D. Although vitamin D is manufactured by the body upon exposure to the correct wavelength of ultraviolet light, and the vitamin D requirement can be met if the skin is adequately exposed to sunlight or artificial ultraviolet light of the correct wavelength, latitude, season, skin pigmentation, age, general health, and cultural practices affect vitamin D synthesis (National Research Council 1989b). Smith (1990) reports that the wavelength of "winter sunlight in northern latitudes is useless for the production of vitamin D. . . . Thus, in Boston (at 42° North . . .) exposure of the skin to such sunlight as exists will not result in any synthesis of vitamin D from between about 1st November to 1st March, and in Glasgow (56° North. . .) matters must be far worse" (900). Women in some cultures cover nearly every part of their bodies even in warm weather; the aged and the ill often spend nearly all of their time indoors. People with darker skin need much longer exposures to light to get the same degree of synthesis as those with lighter skin (Clemens *et al.* 1982). With aging, the capacity for skin synthesis of vitamin D declines, and Webb *et al.* (1988) report that "the capacity of skin to synthesize vitamin D_3 in the elderly is approximately half that of young people" (from National Research Council 1989b). Because so many factors interact to limit skin synthesis of vitamin D, nutritionists consider the vitamin "an essential *dietary* nutrient" (National Research Council 1989b, 93, emphasis added).

In addition, "vitamin D is a recognized promoter of calcium absorption" (National Research Council 1989b, 175), and deficiencies of vitamin D result in rickets among children and osteomalacia in adolescence and adults. Rickets results in a malformation of the skeleton, and osteomalacia is a condition of excessive bone loss that leads to fractures in extreme cases (National Research Council 1989b, 92). Rickets has been reported in both vegetarians and nonvegetarians, but unsupplemented vegan and vegetarian diets are lower in vitamin D than diets that include fatty fish, eggs, and meat.[7] Breast-fed infants are especially vulnerable because "the milk of vegan women who consume no vitamin D-fortified foods or vitamin supplements, or who live in colder parts of the country [that is, of the U.S.], is likely to be especially low in the vitamin" (Dwyer and Loew 1994, 95). Supplementation of milk and other foods with vitamin D is largely responsible for the obliteration of childhood rickets in most of the industrialized world (Sanders and Reddy 1994).

Many vegans adopt the diet for moral, religious, or spiritual reasons (Dwyer 1991, 1993). Very likely, the male physiological ideal is assumed by its leaders. For example, Dagnelie *et al.* (1990) report a high prevalence of rickets in Dutch macrobiotic infants, despite the fact that the "educational level was high and no apparent adverse social circumstances prevailed. . . . Ninety-seven percent of the parents had followed macrobiotic courses and lectures" (202). Many followers of Michio Kushi, the leading teacher of macrobiotic principles, continue to resist dietary supplements and dairy products. However, Dagnelie *et al.* (1990) report that Kushi has changed his dietary recommendations to include fatty fish. Dagnelie *et al.* (1990) note that this improves but does not completely solve the problem of vitamin D and calcium deficiencies in the diet of children. They recommend addition of dairy products and reduction of whole grains. The foregoing suggests that macrobiotic principles were formulated by a "vegan ideal" incorporating the male physiological ideal, since the special needs of women and children were not originally considered and even now are granted only as concessions.

In summary, breastfeeding women and their infants are more vulnerable to vitamin D deficiency than are adult males. Human milk is low in vitamin D even in nonvegetarians (and lower still in vegetarians and vegans), providing less than half the RDA for a six-month-old infant, and all breastfed infants should receive supplementation to bring up the daily dose to 7.5 µg (300 IU) from birth to age six months and 10 µg (400 IU) for infants over six months. The latter RDA continues through age twenty-four years, at which time peak bone mass should have been attained. Basing ethical vegetarianism on an male physiological norm increases the burdens for women and children and fails to treat them as equals.

Calcium. Vegan rejection of dairy products significantly reduces sources of calcium from diet. Most of the concern centers on bone health among women and children.[8] *The American Journal of Clinical Nutrition* devoted a supplement issue in 1991 to reviews of questions about the calcium requirement in the diet of all persons. Continued inadequacy of calcium in the diet is thought to be a major contributing factor to osteoporosis (Dawson-Hughes 1991; Matkovic *et al.* 1979; Rodysill 1987), and milk is still recommended as the best source of calcium: "The calcium in milk and milk products is well-absorbed, whereas that in most plant sources is either poorly or negligibly available" (Allen 1986, 7).

"Negligibly available" means that although chemical tests show a vitamin or mineral such as calcium occurs in plants, it either comes in a form the body cannot use very well or occurs in the presence of other compounds (such as phytates, fiber, cellulose, uronic acids and oxalates in the case of calcium) that prevent its use (Dwyer 1991; Freeland-Graves 1988; Truesdell *et al.* 1984). Osteoporosis is a major concern for post-menopausal women. Osteoporosis is a "metabolic bone disease which results in loss of skeletal mass without alteration in the composition of bone" (Rodysill 1987). With bone loss, fractures may occur, particularly of the hip, forearm, and vertebrae.[9] Women are at much greater risk for this disease than men. Although men are not completely exempt, their generally denser skeletons and testosterone levels prevent its occurrence until quite late in life (Johns Hopkins Medical Institutions 1994c). Rodysill (1987) notes that "twenty-five to fifty percent of women over age sixty have evidence of bone demineralization. . . . Thirty-five to fifty percent of women over age sixty-five will suffer fractures of the distal forearm, vertebral bodies or neck of the femur. Up to thirty-two percent of women will suffer hip fractures by age ninety and sixteen percent of women who suffer hip fractures die during the ensuing three months" (743). "Men lose only about one percent of spinal bone mass a decade after age forty (women lose up to ten percent in the decade after menopause)" (Johns Hopkins Medical Institutions 1994c, 3). Kanis (1993) reports that in Europe the "prevalence of osteoporosis amongst elderly women is six-fold that of men," (10) and the Johns Hopkins Medical Institutions (1994c) report a five-fold prevalence in the United States with twenty percent of all cases occurring in males.

Many reviews of the calcium requirement begin by explaining the process of bone formation and bone loss and the factors associated with it. From the supplement issue above:

> All tissues are involved in growth and none more so than the skeleton. From birth to puberty it increases by about sevenfold and by a further threefold during adolescence. . . . An essential requirement for healthy bone development during childhood and adolescence is a continuous supply of calcium phosphate in amounts regulated to the changing needs of growth. The only source of calcium available to the body is that contained in the diet. . . . Absorption of calcium is not efficient, its bioavailability from the diet is variable, and it is continuously excreted in urine, feces, and sweat as an obligatory loss (Peacock 1991)

Childhood and adolescence are a time to build peak bone mass and the better it is built, the more bone there will be, such that when bone loss begins it will take a longer time to reach a stage of severe depletion. Young women have already built almost all of their bone by about age seventeen with some new bone formation perhaps continuing into the twenties (Dawson-Hughes 1991). By age thirty many women begin to lose bone (Rodysill 1987). Since males have a generally larger bone mass, their incidence of osteoporosis is much lower. For women:

> Over the first several years after menopause, the skeleton undergoes a period of accelerated mineral loss in the process of adapting to declining concentrations of estrogen. After this period of adjustment, the rate of bone loss declines and remains fairly constant (Dawson-Hughes 1991).

Most researchers agree that new bone cannot be built by diet or calcium supplementation after young adulthood, and the best that can be hoped for is arresting or attenuating bone loss.[10] But calcium is important in the slowing of bone loss and consequent postponement of osteoporosis (see Dawson-Hughes' 1991 review of 66 studies).

Adolescent girls who consumed diets low in calcium have been shown to have lower bone mineral density later in life (Peacock 1991; Sandler *et al.* 1985). Sandler *et al.* (1985) questioned 255 Caucasian women aged 49 to 66 years about their lifelong habits of milk consumption. Their data indicate that

> women who reported drinking milk with every meal during childhood and adolescence had significantly higher bone densities than women who reported drinking milk less frequently. . . . The data show a nearly linear relationship between frequency of milk consumption and bone densities. . . . Moreover, when those who reported milk consumption with every meal up to the age of 35 (n = 42) were compared with those who reported rarely consuming milk throughout those years (n = 15), the differences previously noted were magnified. . . . [They] had significantly higher bone densities . . . , indicating that a degree of protection against ABL [accelerated bone loss] was imparted (272–73).

The studies cited in reviews provide good support for a causal relation between higher milk ingestion in adolescence and lower incidence of osteoporosis later in life. In addition, the American Dietetic Association reports that lactovegetarians have a lower incidence of osteoporosis (Havala and Dwyer 1988; see also Freeland-Graves 1988 and Tylavsky and Anderson 1988).

Calcium is the major constituent of bone, but many other factors affect bone health. Lifestyle and other dietary factors that affect bone loss include alcohol and caffeine consumption, physical exercise, and hormone levels.[11] As mentioned above, vitamin D is a promoter of calcium absorption. Calcium deficiencies are seen in those suffering osteomalacia, secondary to vitamin D deficiency (Finch *et al.* 1992). Strause and Saltman (1993) found that post-menopausal women taking the trace elements copper, manganese, and zinc with 1000 mg calcium per day had arrested their bone loss compared to those who took trace elements or calcium alone. These researchers comment: "By eating a reasonable and prudent diet after menopause, women can significantly reduce their risk of osteoporosis. . . . Women who eliminate dairy products, the largest source of Ca [calcium], and red meats, the most bioavailable source of the trace minerals, from their diets are at the greatest risk of nutritional deficiencies. Selection of low-fat dairy products and lean meats will decrease caloric intake without the subsequent loss of nutrients from the diet" (Strause and Saltman 1993, 3).[12] Vegan women are advised by nutritionists to increase their intakes of dietary calcium from plant sources and, if these are insufficient, to take at least 600 mg of elemental calcium daily with meals (Dwyer 1991; Dwyer and Loew 1994).

Even though elderly women suffer osteoporosis to a greater degree than elderly males, the importance of building peak bone mass in adolescence should not be minimized for male adolescents. Because the population is living longer, osteoporosis is becoming more common in elderly men; twenty percent of all cases occur in elderly males in the United States (Johns Hopkins Medical Institutions 1994c).

Elderly persons, whether male or female, with "systemic diseases such as thyroid dysfunction, glucocorticoid excess and hyperparathyroidism" may also suffer osteoporosis, although these etiologies are less common (Rodysill 1987, 743). Medications such as tetracycline, isoniazid, over-the-counter aluminum-containing antacids (such as Amphojel, Gelusil, Maalox), anticonvulsants (such as Dilantin), the diuretic furosemide (Lasix), thyroid hormone, heparin, and systemic or glucocorticoid therapy may accelerate bone loss and lead to osteoporosis (Rodysill 1987; Johns Hopkins Medical Institutions 1994c). About forty percent of the mostly elderly men who have osteoporosis of the spine also have illnesses or take medicines that interfere with calcium absorption (Johns Hopkins Medical Institutions 1994c).

In Western industrialized countries, the loss of estrogen production that accompanies menopause or surgical removal of the ovaries may be the most important factor in accelerated bone loss (Dawson-Hughes 1991). Estrogen replacement (HRT) has been shown to slow bone demineralization and reduce fracture rates (Rodysill 1987). There are increased risk factors for women using

HRT, such as for endometrial and breast cancer, and there are other benefits such as delay of coronary heart disease. However, evaluation of these depends on individual cases. As such, these choices are not open to decision making on the basis of a universal moral principle condemning dairy product consumption.

Thus, using dairy products or supplements is recommended for most women. "Many experts, as well as the National Institutes of Health and the National Osteoporosis Foundation, recommend that postmenopausal women take up to 1,500 mg daily, to compensate for accelerated calcium loss" (Johns Hopkins Medical Institutions 1994b, 5). The efficacy, safety, and environmental impact of supplement use is discussed further on.

The male physiological ideal is sexist, ageist, westernized and industrialized because it presupposes no differences between the sexes and between age groups as well as a safe, adequate, and vitamin and mineral fortified food supply. In other parts of the world, studies have shown similar correlations between calcium intake and bone density. Nordin (1966) compared populations in Finland, the United Kingdom, the United States, Gambia, Jamaica, India, and Japan and noted a striking relationship between osteoporotic x-rays of the spine and low calcium intake and also between high calcium intake and normal vertebral appearance in those countries, especially among females. Even though this study is old, Pollitzer and Anderson (1989) still call it "impressive." Where dairy products are available, women have better bone health. Recently, for instance, Hu *et al.* (1993) report an association between very low intakes of calcium in youth and lower bone density among middle-aged and elderly women in five rural counties in China: "The results strongly indicated that dietary calcium, especially from dairy sources, increased bone mass in middle aged and elderly women by facilitating optimal peak bone mass earlier in life" (219).[13]

NUTRITIONAL VULNERABILITIES FOR LACTOVEGETARIANS

Before I begin to discuss the differences in people on common U.S. diets and those on lactoovovegetarian diets, let me say something about my own thoughts. When I read the research in 1987, my younger daughter was ten years old. My husband and I decided to become vegetarians after reading the arguments of Regan (1983) and Singer (1975). But, I had moral responsibilities concerning my daughter to insure her health as well as to give her a moral education. Should I have withheld milk from her diet because dairying is arguably immoral? What would I say later if she were to develop osteoporosis? Should I have given up milk and cheese in premenopause? Ultimately, my husband and I decided that we should not eat meat but that my daughter's diet should be unrestricted, given

her stage of life. We would restrict but not eliminate dairy products for ourselves. This decision created other kinds of problems: In my family, I am the
person who prepares the food, so the burden of learning new recipes fell entirely
to me. I also prepared different foods for my daughter, although she would
sometimes (but not always) eat what we did. Both she and my husband dislike
vegetables intensely, and there seemed to be very little I could do to change their
dietary preferences. In my experience, ethical vegetarians usually brush off such
concerns as trivial matters of convenience and taste, easily altered by a little education. Yet food preparation is a burden that is disproportionately borne by
women not only in our society but worldwide. Marjorie DeVault's *Feeding the
Family* (1991), a study of thirty families from various social strata and ethnic
groups, illuminates the complexity of the work of feeding family members,
many of whom have different tastes and beliefs. Even in households where the
cooking is shared, a disproportionate share of the labor falls to women (see
63–64). Failure to consider this imbalance of power is also typical of ethical systems that presume a male norm (Sherwin 1989) and stereotypic sex roles. Little
or nothing is said in the arguments for ethical veganism by its proponents to recognize this particular kind of inequality (Singer, 1975; Regan 1983; Pluhar
1992, 1993, 1994; Varner 1994a,b,c).

The moralist claims that children can be taught to like some foods and
reject others, but scientific studies show that "many food preferences appear to
be determined in large part by the genes. Among these are the preferences for
sweet, salt, and milk. The genes also appear responsible, at least to some extent
for . . . the rejection response system for bitter substances" (Logue 1986, 79). In
recent twin studies, "genetic factors were found to influence preference for
orange juice, broccoli, cottage cheese, chicken, sweetened cereal, and hamburger" (Falciglia and Norton 1994, 130). Here, I do not claim genetic deter-
minism. Environmental factors, including education, do play a strong role, of
course, but it is simply not true that foods taste the same to everyone, or that
food preferences are easily or completely amenable to education. Thus, in cases
where genetic taste preferences are strong, parents confront situations of conflict in attempting to teach children to change them. Such battles may precipitate eating dysfunction. Evidence from studies suggests that family conflicts
over food are associated with body image disturbance, lowered self-esteem,
obesity, and eating disorders such as bulimia (see discussion below).

In the end, I could not restrict my daughter's diet because even lactovegetarian diets pose some nutritional risks. These risks are rare for Western adult
males, for whom the ideal is best-suited. Meats provide important sources of

iron and zinc, and adolescents can be picky eaters who are highly resistant to eating the plant foods where these minerals are found.

Iron. The vulnerabilities of women and children to iron deficiency will demonstrate again the adult male, westernized physiological norm that is assumed in the ethical vegetarian arguments. Only a few years ago, marginal iron levels in women were not regarded with much alarm by physicians and nutritionists. Recently, however, it has been found that iron plays a vital role in childhood development and maintenance of the central nervous system, organ function, and immune function (Dallman 1989). Researchers usually categorize their test subjects as "normal," "iron deficient," or "iron deficient anemic," where iron deficiency is a state preceding anemia. In a review of forty-five studies, Hercberg and Galan (1989) note that iron deficiency has "effects on skeletal muscle, cardiac muscle, brain tissue, liver tissue, gastrointestinal tractus [*sic*], body temperature relation, [and] DNA synthesis [because] iron participates in a wide variety of biochemical processes. . . . The key liabilities of tissue iron deficiency, *even at a mild degree* relate to decrease in intellectual performance, and in physical capacity during exercise, alteration of temperature regulation, [and] immune function" (emphasis added, 63). Dallman (1989), in a review of thirty-one studies, notes "there is convincing evidence of impaired psychomotor development and cognitive performance" in iron deficient infants and children (367), and Scrimshaw (1991) cites studies which show that iron deficiency anemia has been associated with irreversible neurological impairment in young children (50; see also Parks and Wharton 1989). Oski 1993 reviews iron deficiency in infancy and childhood and reports:

> An association of iron deficiency during infancy with changes in behavioral development has been shown in at least five separate studies performed in four separate cultures. . . . In all five studies, lower scores on the Bayley mental-development index were observed in the infants with iron-deficiency anemia. The study of Walter *et al.* [1989] reported that performance scores were lower among infants who had had anemia for at least three months than among those who had had anemia for less than three months . . . the reversal of anemic, iron-deficient state did not produce an improvement in the test scores, suggesting the iron-deficiency anemia at a critical period of brain growth and differentiation may produce irreversible abnormalities. . . . Impairment of short-term memory, poor exercise performance, and loss of a sense of well-being have also been reported among iron-deficient adolescents (193).

Thus, the effects of diets without adequate available sources of iron in infancy and young childhood cannot be compensated for by later improvements and/or later supplementation. In addition, "maternal mortality, prenatal and perinatal infant death and prematurity are significantly increased" for iron deficiency in pregnancy (Scrimshaw 1991, 50; see also Dallman 1989).

Milk and other dairy products are poor sources of iron, although what little iron there is in breast milk is better absorbed (up to fifty percent absorbable) than what occurs in cow's milk (up to ten percent absorbable) (Oski 1993). Heme-iron (from meats) "is absorbed regardless of the other components in the diet, while non-haem [*sic*] iron absorption is subject to the interplay of promoting and inhibiting substances in the diet" (Bothwell *et al.* 1989, 357). Heme-iron enhances the absorption of non-heme (plant source) iron, but diets with too many polyphenols and phytates from grains give poor iron absorption (Bothwell *et al.* 1989; Dwyer 1991). This means that eating meat with iron-containing vegetables enhances the absorption of the iron in the vegetables. Eating whole grains (especially wheat) with plant iron *reduces* absorption as does drinking tea (but not coffee). Heme-iron from beef is available in the highest quantities (Scrimshaw 1991, 48). Vitamin C can double absorption of non-heme iron, but this effect is not thought to sufficiently offset the advantages of heme-iron sources (Dwyer and Loew 1994; Oski 1993).

A significant number of women become iron deficient during pregnancy even when they are not vegetarians (Bothwell *et al.* 1989), and nutritionists have expressed concern that because vegetarian diets restrict nutrient sources these diets may not provide adequate iron (Dwyer 1991). Although pregnant "vegan women [in the United States] can meet increased needs for most nutrients during pregnancy by diet alone . . . iron needs rise so much after the second trimester that supplements are usually needed since plant sources of iron are less bioavailable than heme iron" (Dwyer and Loew 1994, 91). The Committee on Maternal Nutrition of the Food and Nutrition Board of the National Academy of Sciences (1990) recommends 30 mg ferrous iron supplementation for all pregnant women in the second and third trimesters, regardless of their diets. Taking higher amounts is not recommended because of interference with other nutrients.

Iron deficiency among women is common around the world. Even "in the United States, Japan, and Europe, . . . between ten and twenty percent of women of childbearing age are anemic" (Scrimshaw 1991, 48). "Nutritional anaemia is recognized as a major public health problem throughout the world, especially in developing countries. . . . Sufficient evidence suggests that iron deficiency is the most common cause of nutritional anaemia in the world" (Hercberg and Galan

1992). The particular sensitivity of women to iron deficiency is related to periodic blood loss at menses and during pregnancy (Scrimshaw 1991; Hercberg and Galan 1992). Unlike calcium, iron is not lost through the urine and only minuscule amounts appear in sweat. Iron loss occurs primarily through bleeding.

Greater incidence and severity of iron deficiency in women and children occur in areas where education about adequate intakes of iron and B_{12} is not available or where the food supply is inadequate or undependable and is four to six times more common in Third World countries than in industrialized countries: "two-thirds of children and women of childbearing age in most developing nations are estimated to suffer from iron deficiency" (Scrimshaw 1991, 48). The anemia is often more severe in developing countries. People in Europe and the United States rarely suffer death, dwarfism, papilledema and subsequent blindness, hypogonadism, or severe pica that accompany severe and chronic iron deficiency anemia (Fairbanks *et al.* 1971). Scrimshaw attributes "poor absorption from the predominantly vegetarian diets of most people in developing countries [as] a primary cause of iron deficiency" (1991, 48). Contributing causes in Third World countries include other disease factors such as parasites; these are not, however, thought to be the sole cause of iron deficiency, since supplementation can improve growth and blood iron levels in anemic children where parasitic infection is common (see Latham *et al.* 1990).

Among United States infants, "iron status usually becomes a problem among exclusively breastfed infants and in infants who are not given iron fortified formula or iron supplements after six months of age. Normal iron status is usually maintained among full term infants up to that point, because liver stores of iron and fetal hemoglobin suffices" (Dwyer and Loew 1994, 96).

In the United States, iron deficiency anemia in children is associated with socioeconomic class. In areas of our country where infants do not get fortified formulas or cereals, studies show a much higher incidence of iron deficiency in young children. Oski (1993) reports a 19.7 percent incidence of iron deficiency and 8.2 percent incidence of iron deficiency anemia among inner-city one-year-old infants who did not receive iron-fortified formula. Infants from the same inner city who participated in infant nutrition programs, such as WIC, had only a one percent incidence of iron deficiency. Vegan infants who are not breastfed should receive "commercial formulas made from soy isolate, which contain methionine, calcium, zinc, iron, riboflavin, vitamin B_{12}, [and] vitamin D" rather than homemade or unfortified soy milk (Dwyer and Loew 1994, 96). The latter do not provide the added vitamins and minerals and may not be heated enough to deactivate the antitrypsin factor which is present in soybeans and inhibits one of the gut enzymes.

In addition, several studies have confirmed depletion of body iron stores in adolescent female athletes (Rowland 1990); supplementation can improve iron status but not endurance (Klingshirn *et al.* 1992). Nieman (1988) reports that "some female athletes may increase their risk of iron deficiency and/or amenor-rhea if a restrictive vegetarian [vegan] diet is adopted" (754).

Evidence from two recent studies also reinforce the claim that iron require-ments differ for males and females and differentially affect health status. Salonen *et al.* (1992) found an increased risk for myocardial infarction [heart attack] in men with high stored-iron levels. In a prospective study of 3,287 men and 5,269 women, Stevens *et al.* (1994) found that moderate elevation of body iron, that is, stored iron, increases the risk of cancer in both men and women,[14] but males are at greater risk because females rarely have elevated iron levels until after menopause. Interestingly, Stevens *et al.* (1994) do not suggest that men curb their intake of such high iron foods as beef, but instead say that while "the results presented here do not weaken or invalidate the considerable evidence of adverse health effects of severe iron deficiency, . . . these data do, however, call into question the wisdom of wholesale addition of iron to food" (368). Since iron fortification of foods has largely benefited women and chil-dren where it has been instituted, I cite this as an example that the debate about dietary requirements often proceeds in male terms: the health of women and children does not seem to be given equal consideration with that given to men.

Zinc. Zinc is another essential element whose requirement varies by age and sex. Zinc occurs in reasonable amounts in plant foods, but as with iron, "flesh foods provide larger, more easily absorbed amounts" (Dwyer and Loew 1994, 93). "Meat, liver, eggs, and seafoods (especially oysters) are good sources of available zinc, whereas whole grain products contain the element in a less avail-able form" (National Research Council 1989b, 207). The reason zinc from whole grains cannot be used as well by the body is that cereals and vegetables contain phytates and fiber that bind zinc chemically, and so it passes through the body unused (Truesdell and Acosta 1985, 838).

Zinc is a component of the enzymes that control protein metabolism, cell replication, and cell differentiation,[15] as well as those enzymes that synthesize DNA (deoxyribonucleic acid) and RNA (ribonucleic acid). As such, zinc is involved in all stages of the cell cycle (Institute of Medicine 1990, 300). Zinc deficiency and the functions of zinc are incompletely understood and have been less fully studied than those of iron and calcium. Dietary deficiency pro-duces loss of appetite, changes in ability to taste, slowed wound healing, slowed growth, skin changes, and abnormalities in immune function (National Research Council 1989b, 206–07). Severe zinc deficiency is rare, but has been observed in the Middle East among men, where dwarfism and hypogonadism (shrunken or undeveloped testicles) were found (Prasad 1982; see also National Research Council 1989b, 207). Severe zinc deficiency in pregnant women, secondary to inherited impaired zinc absorption, produces major obstetrical complications and congenital malformations in the infant (Institute of Medicine 1990, 301). Such inborn errors of metabolism are rare but give scientists clues about effects of mild to moderate zinc deficiency. It is not clear whether mild zinc deficiencies are a cause of permanent developmental damage. Hambidge et al. (1972) did find "suboptimal growth, poor appetite, and impaired taste acuity" in children with marginal zinc deficiency. They were able to improve these conditions with a small dose of zinc supplementation.

In adolescent vegetarians, zinc intake may be marginal. Jacobs and Dwyer (1988) comment that "in our opinion it is extremely difficult, if not impossible, to consistently meet Zn RDA [zinc recommended daily allowance] on an unsupplemented vegan or even lactoovovegetarian diet" (816). Bakan *et al.* (1993) note that "anorexia nervosa and zinc deficiency, found most frequently in young females, have a number of symptoms in common. These include weight loss, alterations in taste and appetite, depression, and amenorrhea. Approximately half of anorexia nervosa patients are vegetarian, a practice that may increase their risk for zinc deficiency" (229). From the fact that half of these patients are vegetarians who are low or marginal for zinc intake we cannot say that zinc deficiency or vegetarianism is a cause of anorexia nervosa, but the observation is a correlation that is under study.

The foregoing nutritional research shows important differences in the nutritional needs of many women, most children, and elderly persons. Research that showed safety and benefits of vegan or vegetarian diets accrues mostly to Western males. Women and children are known to have more problems on such diets unless they are carefully monitored. Scientifically, no single physiological norm obtains. But the pattern of research may suggest that women and children are treated as outliers, exceptions, and "vulnerable groups," who do not fit expected norms. And certainly, the moralists discussed here claim that anyone can be an ethical vegetarian with no extra special burden. But women and children and some aging people do not fit that male norm. Yet, these people comprise the majority and when cultural, class, and inherited conditions are also considered, that majority becomes vast because it includes a large number of males in the Third World as well.

THE CULTURAL NORM OF WEALTH

Cultures where vegan and lactoovovegetarian diets are a healthy alternative pre-suppose access to health care, literacy, and a stable food supply; that is, wealth.

CULTURAL AND CLASS DIFFERENCES

The "male physiological ideal" also includes bias with respect to culture and class. Priyani Soysa reviews the nutritional status of women in developing coun-tries and comments that the dietary requirements for adult women recom-mended by the Food and Agriculture Organization/World Health Organization (FAO/WHO) refer largely to the industrialized countries and "would not be rel-evant for women in the developing world" (Soysa 1987, 17). Deficiencies in diet are associated with poverty, discrimination against women, inadequate caloric intake, anorexia secondary to parasitic infection and stress from other infections, plus heavy physical workloads (Soysa 1987, 17).

Sometimes vegetarians point to India, where many persons live on largely unsupplemented vegetarian diets, as a place where such diets are possible with-out wealth. But certainly, the Indian subcontinent cannot be cited as a society whose majority are healthy or have enough to eat. The relationship between unsupplemented vegetarian diets and overall life expectancy is far from clear, but ethical vegetarians often buttress their moral arguments with appeals to the health benefits of vegetarian diets, especially as effective in preventing such dis-eases of old age as hypertension and heart disease. Presumably, ethical vegetari-ans believe that life expectancy is likely to be lengthened (although researchers do not make such claims; see Dwyer 1988). For what it is worth, then, we can note that life expectancy in India for females is 55.67 years and for males 55.40 years (United Nations 1991).[16] In India, most people do not live long enough to suffer diseases of old age. Also, in a study of pregnant women and their new-borns in Udaipur, India, Sharma *et al.* conclude that "vegetarianism may be one of the important causative factor [*sic*] of anaemia in pregnant women in this region and their newborn children" (1991, 13). As mentioned above, iron defi-ciency anemia in U.S. children is associated with poverty (Oski 1993), and such anemias are also associated with higher prenatal and infant mortality. Thus, the "norm" is class- and culture-biased.

INHERITED DIFFERENCES

Likewise, the male physiological norm is ethnically biased. Scientists know that diet alone cannot account for the differences in predispositions to develop certain diseases that exist among different ethnic groups due to genetic inheritance. Vegan and vegetarian diets are likely to have different effects on different ethnic groups, thus creating different burdens for ethnic groups to bear in altering their diets to meet the vegan ideal. Genetic factors are known to affect nutrition and to interact with diet in the etiology of certain conditions and disease processes, notably coronary heart disease, hypertension, diabetes mellitus, obesity, cancer, lactose adsorption and malabsorption, and probably others (National Research Council 1989a).[17]

Of particular note: Japanese women have a higher incidence of osteoporosis than Caucasian women, whereas the incidence among Black women is lower than for either group (Pollitzer and Anderson 1989). Researchers believe that these and other differences are associated with inherited differences in the ability to build skeletal mass (see Pollitzer and Anderson 1989).

Although long-term vegetarian diets lowered blood pressure in studied populations of both older whites and older Blacks, Blacks still had "significantly higher average BP [blood pressure] than either dietary group of [vegetarian and nonvegetarian] older white adults" (Melby *et al.* 1993). Blacks apparently have an inherited greater susceptibility to elevation in blood pressure (Melby *et al.* 1993). However, if ethnic differences affect health for ethical vegans, the traditional ethical vegetarian moralist simply grants them excuses. This, too, is objectionable, as I will discuss in a later section.

COUNTERBALANCING CONSIDERATIONS

Ethical vegetarians sometimes claim that vegetarian diets are healthier than any diet containing any meat, eggs, or dairy products (see Pluhar 1992, 1993). Supplementation, they claim, compensates for any differences and deficiencies (see Varner 1994a). Are these counterbalancing considerations sufficient to forget about the bias I have pointed out?

SUPPLEMENTATION

Even in our society, because vegan diets restrict food sources of certain important vitamins and minerals, vegan women and children should probably be taking a variety of supplements depending on their age and whether they are pregnant or lactating. First, even if we agree that supplements and fortified foods do an adequate or even an excellent job of making up for dietary deficiencies, the imperative to supplementation and fortification carries with it several presuppositions, including: (1) supplements are virtually risk-free, (2) supplements work as well as food, (3) those most at risk will take (and receive) supplements,

(4) little or no education is required to use supplements, (5) good education guarantees wise use of supplements, (6) substituting supplements for food will not pose unequal health benefits or burdens on individuals because of their sex, age, race, ethnicity, class, or culture, and (7) broad adoption of supplement use has no serious environmental impacts. There may be other assumptions as well, but I shall not explore them here. All of the presuppositions above are false.

Regarding (1) and (2) above, supplementation, especially for multiple dietary requirements, carries significant risks because of the possibility of low bioavailability, toxicity, and interactions among supplements. Foods produce fewer problems of interaction and availability and rarely, if ever, cause toxicities for the vitamins and minerals cited here. But, where supplements are concerned, our bodies can use some chemical formulations of them better than others. Some supplements may not get into the system where needed at all (for example, see section on *Vitamin B_{12}*), whereas others are well absorbed (Allen 1986; Herbert 1988; Scrimshaw 1991). Some supplements cause side-effects even at RDA levels. For example, iron supplements often cause constipation (Ossell 1993). At RDA levels, supplements are safe and do protect against serious consequences of deficiency, such as rickets and osteomalacia (in vitamin D deficiency), megaloblastic anemia (in vitamin B_{12} deficiency), osteoporosis (in calcium deficiency), and iron deficiency anemia. But, toxicities can occur by taking too much of a supplement and also by taking two or more different kinds of supplement that interact to give a bad reaction. For instance, vitamin D is toxic at high doses as are zinc and iron (National Research Council 1989b). So, it is simply not true that using supplements is risk-free.

Will those most at risk actually take their supplements (3)? Rather than looking at what people should do (from the standpoint of a middle-class college student or professor), look at what they actually do. Motivations are vast and complex and exist in a cultural milieu. For example, although calcium supplementation is often prescribed for perimenopausal women to prevent osteoporosis, the most critical time for calcium consumption appears to be during childhood, adolescence, and young womanhood (Peacock 1991), when bone mass is being built. Nevertheless, according to a review of recent polls on vitamin and mineral usage in the United States, adolescents are among the least likely to take supplements (McDonald 1986)! In addition, many vegans eschew supplementation, often on moral or quasi-moral grounds that arise out of (patriarchal) religious beliefs (Dwyer 1991; Dagnelie *et al.* 1990), and as I noted above, some of these may also incorporate a "vegan ideal" that is modeled on the male body in their dietary prescriptions and refusal of supplementation (such as Kushi macrobiotic diets).

The third presupposition is false on economic grounds as well. Supplements cost money. In a capitalist economy without equal access to health care or work, some socioeconomic classes are simply unable to afford supplements (or food) for their children and consequently nutritional deficiencies arise (Oski 1993; Kozol 1988). Rachel and her children, Mr. Alessandro, his children, and aging mother do not, cannot take or receive supplements, although doubtless they could use them.

As for (4), choosing the right supplement requires some rather sophisticated knowledge. For instance, calcium citrate is recommended to older adults because it is easier to digest, but anyone "with a history of kidney stones should probably avoid citrate-based supplements, since they may be associated with kidney stone formation in susceptible patients" (Johns Hopkins Medical Institutions 1994, 5). Also, in 1982 the Food and Drug Administration (FDA) issued warnings about lead and other heavy metals that are present in calcium supplements (FDA 1982; Liebman 1993). Lead harms the nervous system in children and unborn fetuses and babies. Iron deficiency also increases lead absorption and increases the risk of elevated blood lead concentrations (Dallman 1993). In 1991, the FDA "warned that children aged six and younger should consume no more than six micrograms of lead a day" (Liebman 1993). Bourgoin et al. (1993) analyzed the lead content in seventy brands of calcium tablets sold in the United States and Canada. The lead content varied with the source from which the calcium was derived. When lead ingestion rates based on suggested intakes were calculated, all supplements actually delivered several times the lead level as milk and some up to four or five times the 6 µg "tolerable daily intake for children aged 0–6 years" (see Bourgoin et al. 1993, 1158, fig. 1).[18]

Infants and children with milk allergies often take calcium supplements that may contain lead. Soy-based formulas, soy milk, and other foods are calcium fortified, and the source of the calcium is not known and depends on the manufacturer. The National Center for Health Statistics found that twenty-five percent of U.S. women and eight percent of U.S. children age two to six years take calcium supplements (Moss et al. 1989). Bourgoin et al. (1993) also expressed concern for women age fifty and over, some of whom take 1,000 to 2,000 mg of calcium every day to reduce risk of osteoporosis.[19]

Knowledge of mineral interactions is needed, too. Ingestion of improper amounts of some minerals adversely affects absorption of others; for instance, taking too much iron can result in a zinc deficiency, but taking zinc can upset copper balance (Dwyer 1991; Festa et al. 1985; McDonald and Keen 1988). Pregnant vegan women are advised not to exceed 30 mg ferrous iron per day since vegans and vegetarians tend to have low zinc intakes, and "high doses of iron may depress serum zinc levels" (Dwyer and Loew 1994, 11). Solomons and Jacob (1981) confirm this interaction and also found that the effect did not occur when heme-iron (from meat) or a food source of zinc was substituted. Calcium interacts with vitamin D, aluminum, boron, phosphorus, copper, zinc, manganese and other elements that are essential to its absorption (McDonald and Keen 1988; Strause and Saltman 1993). Vitamin B_{12} may be inactivated by high doses of vitamin C (National Nutrition Consortium, Inc. 1978), although taking vitamin C enhances absorption of non-heme (plant) iron (Dwyer 1991). Supplements cannot substitute for food, and nutritionists recommend that all people obtain their nutrient needs from a variety of foods rather than from supplements (Council on Scientific Affairs 1987).

As for assumption (5)—that good education will promote wise use of supplements—RDAs have been set to minimize or eliminate risk of toxicities and interactions, but the general public is often ignorant of the enormous amount of research and concern that is invested in these recommendations. Incredibly, the higher one's level of education, the more likely people are to take too many supplements (McDonald 1986). Victor Herbert (1980), a well-known researcher on the biochemistry and metabolism of vitamin B_{12} and critic of health quackery, reports that studies show that many people take megadoses of vitamins, hoping to ward off illness or age, even though toxic side-effects of megadosing are well-documented (123–26). Elderly people and those with incurable diseases are apparently especially vulnerable to overuse of supplements (Hartz and Blumberg 1986; McDonald 1986). Herbert and Subak-Sharpe (1990) note that ingestion of iron medication causes several accidental and often fatal poisonings in children every year. Although rare, iron toxicity can cause hemosiderosis in adults, a serious liver disease (Scrimshaw 1991). McDonald (1986) summarizes concerns about overuse:

> Supplement use is often inappropriate, is more common among females than males in almost every age group, is higher in the western part of the United States than in other regions of the country, is higher in whites than in Blacks, and tends to increase with higher education and income. Some segments of the public consume supplemental nutrients at extremely high levels, giving cause for concern about potential toxic effects (27).

The market availability of such supplements also presupposes the influence of an industrialized food process and a sophisticated medical and nutritional understanding by policymakers and consumers—in other words a wealthy industrialized society with its attendant environmental impacts.

Assumption (6) is blatantly false. Substituting supplements for food does place unequal burdens and benefits on individuals simply because of their age, sex, race, ethnicity, class, or culture. The unequal burdens placed on women and children of substituting supplementation are most apparent. Although women are not pregnant and nursing all of their lives, the majority of women alive today have or will have some children. Because women usually remain capable of child-bearing for most of their adult lives, women may have different nutrient needs than men even when they are not gestating or lactating.[20] The best example is that of female adolescents who must take greater care to build bone mass to avoid osteoporosis later. Vegan and lactoovovegetarian diets impose a disproportionate burden on women, children, the elderly, and others, and cannot be said to involve "equal distribution" of nutrients to all. From an economic standpoint, the fact that many vegan women must take such supplements imposes a financial burden on them that adult males are not required to bear.

The assumption that broad adoption of supplements has no serious environmental impacts (7) is discussed below in "The Ecofeminist's Dilemma." Now I wish to take up the second "counterbalancing claim"—the health benefits of vegan and vegetarian diets.

HEALTH BENEFITS

As mentioned earlier, defenders of the vegan ideal point to long-term studies of American and European lactoovovegetarians that demonstrate several health benefits including reduction in blood pressure and reduced risk of cancer (Dwyer 1988; see also chapter 1). There are several reasons to think this research does not override the bias towards males and industrialized culture.

The studies may suggest that males benefit more than women and children in the trade-off of risks and benefits. With respect to heart disease, although women may benefit from the reduction in fat consumption that can accompany vegetarian or vegan diets,[21] men are likely to benefit more because high levels of estrogen often protect middle-age women.[22] For example, Fraser (1988) reviews several studies of Seventh-Day Adventist populations. The data show "lower risk for IHD [ischemic heart disease] in Adventist men . . . probably related to their [mostly lactoovovegetarian] habits, nonsmoking status, possibly their better exercise habits, and greater social support. . . . Similar data for women are somewhat conflicting" (1988, 833).

We also do not know whether ethical vegetarian diets will benefit women on balance. The high-fiber diets (particularly including wheat-bran) recommended to most vegetarians have been correlated with a drop in estrogen levels in women (Rose *et al.* 1991). This would be good for victims of breast cancer, but estrogen decline is also associated with bone loss and osteoporosis (Dawson-Hughes 1991; Rodysill 1987) and might result in increased risk of coronary heart disease in women (Barrett-Connor and Bush 1991).

We do not have a clear idea about the relation of diet and disease in women because nearly all the research has been done on men by male research scientists. Researchers usually rationalize that they assume women will be similarly affected (on the principle of similarity and thus physiological interchangeability), but contradict this claim with the additional rationalization that including women would skew the results by adding the variable of hormonal differences (Ames *et al.* 1990). In July 1991, two studies showed that "although heart diseases kill more than 250,000 American women every year, . . . women are not diagnosed or treated as aggressively as men" (Holloway and Yam 1992, 13). In 1991, the American Medical Association reviewed the studies that show gender disparities in clinical decision making in the treatment of heart disease, kidney disease, and lung cancer; it advised its members to re-evaluate their practice and approach to women's health care (McMurray 1991).[23] Middle-aged men more often die of heart disease; the predominance of white men in government, funding agencies, and the sciences can lead them to focus on problems they are more likely to experience. As Evelyn Fox Keller remarks in a review of masculine biases in science, "presumably had the concerns of medical research been articulated by women, these particular imbalances would not have arisen" (1982, 590).

Vegetarian diets appeal to men's self-interest because these diets can be quite low in fat and may reduce men's incidence of heart disease. Although powerful lobbies continue to press for meat consumption, the power struggle takes place on male terms. The debate entirely overlooks possible differences in the effects of wholesale adoption of restrictive dietary practices (whether they be all-plant or heavily dependent upon meat consumption) on women and children, as well as people of color, old people, and people living in other cultures.[24]

DISCRIMINATION AND THE
PREDICATION OF FIXED NORMS

THE MALE PHYSIOLOGICAL IDEAL

The presumption of a male ideal pervades both nutritional science and moral argument: women, children, and others are referred to in the scientific literature as "nutritionally vulnerable" with respect to certain vitamins and minerals such as iron, calcium, vitamin D, and zinc. All current arguments for ethical vegetarianism treat such "nutritional vulnerability" as an *exception* rather than as a norm. The norm is defined by the adult male body, which is less vulnerable to the adverse health consequences of vegetarian diets. The hidden assumption in the moral arguments is that *being less vulnerable is good*, simply because one is *physically stronger*, and *being more vulnerable is bad* or, at least not as good, because one is *physically weaker*. But that is a bald argument for power rather than for justice, moral virtue, or caring.

Looking at the nutritional evidence, the best candidates for vegetarianism and for veganism, in particular, are young, adult, healthy males living in industrialized cultures. They do not have protein, vitamin, or mineral stresses from feeding a rapidly growing fetus or a nursing infant, nor are they unduly stressed by their own growth requirements, as most of their growth is accomplished. Males have generally larger skeletons and higher iron levels than females and are at much less risk of anemia in adolescence and adulthood and osteoporosis in late middle and old age.

Yet, ethical vegans lobby for universal all-plant diets. They assume that almost every person put in the right set of environmental circumstances (which must include cultural and political settings as well as purely physical ones) could be happy and healthy on vegan diets. They assume that these circumstances can be changed by human choices and, further, that such changes assume no important discrimination against any group and will make the world better rather than worse. But, the assumption that humans can be healthy on vegan diets posits a paradigmatic "normal" human as an adult male herbivore. It ignores any and all differences of biological constitution, especially those that are genetically inherited, whether attributable to sex determination or ethnicity. In contrast, scientists are beginning to find that inherited differences in metabolism are correlated with health and well-being or failure to thrive in alternative environments and circumstances. Real people are not interchangeable with a presupposed "ideal human."[25]

EXCEPTIONS TO THE RULE

To be fair, those defending vegetarianism from traditional moral theories would say that anyone who needs to eat milk, eggs, or meat should not be required to abstain.[26] But all of them argue that these persons will be *exceptional cases*, which can be interpreted to imply that such people will fall outside a stereotypic or fixed physiological norm. Even Regan's (1983) abolitionist animal rights position allows certain persons to consume meat as exceptional cases (333). He says that any humans having a strong welfare-interest in consuming meat or animal products would be *excused* from a duty to be vegetarians. But Regan clearly thinks most people do not or would not (ideally) fall into such a category. He can only assume this if he also assumes that there is a paradigm "normal" human physiology. Women, children, and others who do not fit the norm are excused whenever they have different requirements. But this structure of ethical thinking degrades the reality of these people and reinforces patriarchy with its logic of domination.

Making judgments from the perspective of having a male body about whether people can reasonably choose to be vegetarians and excusing the others is quite unfair. From a white middle-class college professor's perspective, American or Western society may appear quite homogeneous. The education level is high, food is available in great variety, is plentiful and fortified, the unemployed have food stamps, supplements seem readily available.[27] These are conditions of great wealth by world standards. These are the conditions that make veganism reasonably safe. But as the vignette at the beginning of the book shows, simply living in the United States does not guarantee these conditions. American society is a bundle of many cultures and heritages uprooted from their indigenous surroundings.[28] A significant number of Americans do not have access to adequate food or nutritional information, and they are defined by their economic class. Rachel, Mr. Alessandro, and the people who live in the Hotel Martinique cannot buy vegetables—there is no supermarket nearby (Kozol 1988). Shall we simply excuse them then? But there really is something quite arrogant about excusing all of these people from attaining the ideal; it supposes the richer are better. They are not. They are just luckier.

THE PROBLEM WITH EXCUSES—GENDER AND CLASS BIAS

Who are these others that traditionalists like Regan think may be excused? They are the vast majority of the *world's* population. And, if women, and infants, and children, and the elderly, and those who live almost everywhere else besides Western societies are *routinely* excused for doing what would normally be considered wrong, in practice, this relegates them to a *moral underclass* of beings who, because of their natures or cultures, are not capable of being fully moral. They are *physiologically* barred from "doing the right thing" because they are not "being the right thing."

I have shown that risks and burdens for women and men, the old and the young, and those of different races, ethnicities, and classes differ on vegetarian diets. Yet, risk is not the primary issue. The main issue is this: From whose perspective and context shall we assess risk? From the perspective of largely white, relatively affluent adult Western males? Or from the perspective of women or their children? From the context of a high-tech society or that of the so-called Third World?

If the main concern were about risk, advocates for animal rights such as Regan could simply respond that, if women need milk or meat, they have a valid moral excuse (based on the Liberty Principle) from a duty not to kill or harm animals. Women whose health would be jeopardized or whose fetuses would be injured are excused from a duty to make themselves worse off for the sake of another. What ethical vegan/vegetarians fail to see is that a male norm is assumed, and all other body types are assigned a secondary place. The perspectival bias is especially apparent when we consider the position of many Third World women and children, whose unsupplemented food sources and paucity of medical care make a vegan diet much more likely to compromise health. The privileges of wealth form a nexus within which a vegan lifestyle becomes a *healthy alternative*. Vegans must supplement their diets with certain vitamins, especially B_{12} and D, and infants, children, women and others may need supplementation for certain minerals, especially calcium, iron, and zinc (Dwyer 1991). The continued understanding of differences in nutritional requirements among women and men at various stages of life and of various ethnic/genetic ancestry presupposes a sophisticated research scientific and industrial complex. For example, it presupposes the existence of vitamin and mineral factories with the ability to synthesize supplements without using animal products. For that, research biochemistry and chemistry labs are necessary, mines for extraction of raw materials, and a network of universities to train scientists, and so forth. When women, children, and the less privileged are routinely excused for doing what would normally be considered wrong (eating meat, say), they are judged less capable of being fully moral. Likewise when all those people who live in environments that are rural, migratory, marginal, tropical, arctic, alpine, arid, oceanic, isolated or otherwise non-industrialized and largely nonarable are routinely excused, they, too, are judged less capable of full morality.

We live in a global community. We need to know how to treat humans and animals all over the world. As it is now, there is ethnocentric bias in the vegan ideal. It presupposes power. It entwines power with a false virtue. When nearly everyone on Earth, except the most privileged class of humans, is excused from living the most virtuous life on grounds that their natures or their cultures bar them from this, we should suspect that the moral tradition itself has been set up to serve that class and that class alone. We should suspect that we need a better ethical theory.

THE LOGIC OF DOMINATION

Failure to accord equal value to various physiologico-cultural perspectives builds the logic of domination into ethical vegetarianism by setting up the conditions of unwarranted guilt and lowered self-esteem. In some future vegan (or even lactoovovegetarian) world, even if the "excused classes" felt rationally justified in consuming meat or animal products, these people would nevertheless suffer feelings of responsibility for the associated evil—just as a person who kills in self-defense still feels responsible even if not culpable for a killing. Additionally, in a vegan world, even if some people were to consume animal products for health reasons, they would probably suffer social condemnation—largely because we do not ordinarily know the reasons for a stranger's actions. Perhaps such individuals could be issued armbands or other marks designating their status as "excused." In that case, though, it is hard to avoid the conclusion that they would be regarded as abnormal at best or pariahs at worst. Because traditional moral arguments for ethical vegetarianism presuppose this logic of domination, they cannot be incorporated into ecofeminist arguments for vegetarianism. Nor will it be sufficient simply to "add a little feeling and emotion" to a supposedly too sterile, but essentially correct moral argument for animal welfare and animal rights. The presuppositions of the arguments, whether moral sentiments are added or not, are themselves discriminatory.

THE UNACCEPTABLE FEMALE BODY

Some of the most important work in feminist theory has been scholarship that reclaims the embodied image of woman as woman. Women's bodies have been deemed unacceptable in a variety of ways in so many cultures that recounting only a few examples will be possible here. Women have been expected to endure painful and dangerous alterations to virtually every part of their bodies to conform with cultural expectations. Outright mutilations offer clear examples. Done ostensibly to make the female more acceptable to the male, these alterations restrict the woman's power and physically enslave her to the male. Andrea Dworkin (1974) uses the example of footbinding to illustrate the relation of body image to restrictions on freedom and then compares the salient features of the practice to Western ideals of beauty. Footbinding literally made women unable to walk, but today's expectations limit women psychologically as well:

"Standards of beauty describe in precise terms the relationship that an individual will have to her own body. They prescribe her mobility, spontaneity, posture, gait, the uses to which she can put her body. *They define precisely the dimensions of her physical freedom.* And, of course, the relationship between physical freedom and psychological development, intellectual possibility, and creative potential is an umbilical one.

"In our culture, not one part of a woman's body is left untouched, unaltered. No feature or extremity is spared the art, or pain, of improvement. Hair is dyed, lacquered, straightened, permanented; eyebrows are plucked, penciled, dyed; eyes are lined, mascaraed, shadowed; lashes are curled, or false—from head to toe, every feature of a woman's face, every section of her body, is subject to modification, alteration. . . . From the age of eleven or twelve until she dies, a woman will spend a large part of her time, money, and energy on binding, plucking, painting, and deodorizing herself" (Dworkin 1974, 217).

The impetus to dieting and plastic surgery to achieve the "Barbie doll" image pervades our culture and sends the message to ordinary women that their personal worth depends upon their being blonde, incredibly slim, and extraordinarily buxom. Preoccupations with activities to measure up to such physiological goals divert women from participating in other avenues of power. Women define themselves as "good" in relation to how well they match the Barbie ideal, and the vast majority of American women are dissatisfied with their weight, even if it is within normal range. Dieting is practically universal. Culture teaches women to accept a norm for their bodies that is medically unhealthy, but the norm is not one a rational woman would accept in a women-only society. That is, if women were defining the norm apart from perceived male expectations, the female physiological ideal would look different and her attitudes toward food would be healthier.[29] She would perhaps be less afflicted with self-destructive responses to food.

EATING DISORDERS AND MORAL GOODNESS

Barbie is anorexic too. Analysis of the body structure of the doll by Yale professor Kelly Brownell (1995, 1998) indicates that "a 5-foot-2-inch woman weighing 125 pounds would have to grow two feet taller, add five inches to her chest and lose six inches from her waist to look like Barbie . . . 'If healthy, normal-weight individuals use such models as standards for comparison, discontent is a logical outcome. Despair may be the outcome with people who weigh more,' says Professor Brownell.[30] "Anorexia nervosa affects about one percent of women between the ages of twelve and forty" (Brotman 1994, 8). In 1985, the newsletter of the American Anorexia and Bulimia Association reported that these disorders "strike a million Americans every year and that one hundred fifty thousand die annually" (reported in Brumberg 1988, 19–20). A recent textbook on abnormal psychology reports that anorexia nervosa and bulimia nervosa[31] have risen to epidemic proportions, with the number of cases in some areas quadrupling in the time period between 1956 and 1975 (Barlow and Durand 1995). "This epidemic would be puzzling enough if it were occurring across the population as a whole. What makes it more intriguing is that anorexia and bulimia are highly culturally specific" (Barlow and Durand 1995, 299–300). These disorders occur only in the Western world and "over ninety percent of the cases of severe eating disorders are found in young, white females of upper socioeconomic status who are living in a competitive environment" (300). The American Psychiatric Association recently classified these eating disorders as a separate group in DSM–IV. The exact causes of anorexia nervosa are unknown, but all researchers note that social expectations of women that meld personal worth, moral worth, and diet become a toxic brew for some young women or a long-term, low grade self-destructive pattern for others. Psychologists attribute eating disorders among Western women to the "emphasis on appearance, sociocultural standards of beauty and weight, and the changing status and roles of women" (Probart and Lieberman 1992, 151). Adolescent women are particularly vulnerable to dieting, body image disturbance, and lowered self-esteem. Women with eating disorders have often felt pressured to be thin in order to succeed and may start dieting as young as age eleven. Eating is associated with feelings of guilt. In any competitive environment where smallness is advantageous, such as gymnastics, modeling, ballet and other forms of dance, figure skating, crew, and others, young women are more vulnerable. The feminine ideal body weight has declined significantly since 1960 so that in 1992 "sixty-nine percent of the *Playboy* centerfolds and sixty percent of the Miss America contestants had weights fifteen percent or more *below* their expected weights for their age and height. Being this much underweight actually meets one of the criteria for anorexia" (Barlow and Durand 1995, 313).

Anorexia nervosa is usually classified as an illness today, whereas refusal of food and a mystic ability to survive without eating in medieval through nineteenth century times was often looked upon as a sign of spiritual power. The media "discovered" eating disorders about ten years ago, but aberrant eating patterns have been classed as illness by medicine for three centuries and have been recorded since ancient times (Pertschuk 1993). Rudolph Bell (1985) and Caroline Walker Bynum (1987) analyzed the histories of women saints from the High Middle Ages, and "where writings by these women survive, we find the same pervasive images of eating, drinking, and food that appear in the thought of the twentieth-century anorectic who is food obsessed, constantly counts calories, and structures her life around the avoidance of food" (Brumberg 1988, 2). Joan

Jacobs Brumberg argues that such behaviors among medieval women are not properly labeled "anorexia nervosa." Food-refusing behaviors have been subject to varying interpretations in society, and the women themselves offered different reasons for it. Brumberg (1988) examines the cases of nineteenth century "fasting girls" in England and America and compares them with cases from the sixteenth century. She argues that our "understanding of food-refusing behavior evolved in response to new developments in religion and medicine" (4). Interpretation of these behaviors evolved from "sainthood to patienthood" via "secularization and medicalization" (4).

The main point is that for centuries women have associated moral goodness and personal acceptability with ability to forego food. Today, the woman of power is the woman who can "just say no" to food. But, as Brumberg notes, "culture is the critical variable that explains why and how anorexia nervosa became the characteristic psychopathology of the female adolescent of our day. . . . The disease starkly illustrates the predicament of the privileged but vulnerable adolescent female in a rapidly changing society that elevates thinness to the *highest moral plane*. From the vantage point of the historian, anorexia nervosa appears to be a secular addiction to a new kind of perfectionism, one that links personal salvation to the achievement of an external body configuration rather than an internal spiritual state" (Brumberg 1988, 7; emphasis added).

Associations of food with guilt are common—think of the "sinfulness" of chocolate and other rich desserts. As food preparers, women more commonly give up food in order that their husbands and children may eat. The attitude that "an ideal woman [wife] is one who is satisfied with little and is capable of any kind of self-sacrifice" is taught as a virtue in cultures all over the world (see Rizvi 1991, 106). Barlow and Durand (1995) report that "some anorexic individuals, perhaps as a demonstration of absolute control over their eating, show increased interest in cooking and food. Some have become expert chefs, preparing all of the food for the family" (306). Morag MacSween (1993) finds anorexia nervosa to be "one of a range of 'solutions' to the irreconcilability of individuality and femininity [and] one engagement with the dilemmas of patriarchy" (255). But the effort is futile because the only self that can exist in patriarchal culture is the masculine self—the individualized and atomistic self that is antithetical to women's receptive psychology, which is itself the result of social control of women rather than a failure of individual development:

> Anorexic transformation . . . is an individual transformation of social meaning; what the anorexic woman struggles to contain is not her own appetite but feminine desire. The individual woman cannot negate social meaning; in the end it comes to control her,

> either as appetite or as denial . . . she can never in her single body
> deny enough or be thin enough to contain its threat. This, then, is
> the 'moral spiral' . . . of anorexia. She continues to elaborate her
> rituals of denial in a never ending spiral, and never finally and
> securely reaches the place where, with personal control of her body
> as an object, she could begin to act as a subject (250).

MacSween's conclusion is that autonomy and femininity are irreconcilable. Therefore, simply teaching the anorexic female that autonomy is both possible and acceptable will only deny the reality of what the anorexic woman feels. In my interpretation, such attempts would resubmerge these women into patriarchy and participate in the logic of domination. MacSween argues that it is not simply "outdated and faulty upbringing" that predisposes some young girls to anorexia. It is rather the "social control of women" within the structures of social meaning and social practices that negates the reality of the feminine.

In the "logic of denial" affirmed by MacSween (1993) in the quotations from patients, "the anorexic body is empty inside, and emptiness means being clean. It is not contaminated by external things, but is *pure*" (248; emphasis added). If MacSween's exposition is valid, the social meaning that connects impurity with some kinds of food (see Twigg's 1979 essay on purity and vegetarianism summarized in the previous chapter) has been intensified in the anorectic to count all food as impure and so as an assault on her virtue, her goodness, her moral character. A good girl is a thin girl.

Nutritionists and researchers believe that associating moral guilt with food is a contributing factor in eating disorders and have warned against teaching these ideas to children and adolescents (Tufts University 1993). Thus, claims about the immorality of eating meat or consuming dairy products may exacerbate the vulnerability of young women to anorectic behaviors. Feminism cannot endorse anorectic or bulimic responses as authentic expressions of feminine power and self-determination. Rather, eating disorders are the manifestations of our oppression. Telling us that "good girls don't eat meat" will very likely exacerbate our oppression rather than relieve it.

THE ECOFEMINIST'S DILEMMA

Ecofeminists reject the universality in traditional moral theory and its "logic of domination" that has governed the mechanization of culture and the instrumentalization of nature (Warren 1990). They reject the misuse and overuse of technology and often attack Western medicine and science. "Development" in the Third World has often meant exacerbating the exploitation of women and animals (Shiva 1989). They call for us to "*see* the tree; but . . . also the logging industry . . . the downed cow in the slaughterhouse pen . . . but also see the farming and dairy industry . . ." (Donovan 1996). They emphasize the necessity of extensive contextual and political analysis of ethical questions. In this section, I outline such a political analysis of arguing for the ethical vegetarian life.

Ecofeminist Carol Adams (1993) specifically rejects the claim of people from other cultures to eating animals and their products, claiming humans have no need of them. But, if people and animals are equal, the implication is that technology and supplementation *must* be taken to the Third World.

Much of our food is highly processed and fortified. We tend to think of our food as "naturally" protecting us. And it does! Even the worst junk food diet is unlikely to result in pellagra or beriberi in the United States because virtually all flours are vitamin B fortified. Vitamin D is added to milk and is perhaps the single most important factor in the reduction of the incidence of rickets in children and osteomalacia in women and adolescents (Sanders and Reddy 1994).

In the many parts of the world, beriberi, pellagra, rickets, scurvy, kwashikor, megaloblastic anemia, and iron deficiency are still endemic (Scrimshaw 1990),[32] although the incidence has declined this century and the severity of the affected is usually less marked. Americans are so well-fed that we take it for granted that our foods will protect us against these diseases, but that protection depends on food preservation, rapid transportation, fortification, variety and plenty.

Vegan and vegetarian diets are safe in Western nations when individuals have access to education, medical care, and sufficient resources to buy proper foods. And these diets pose less risk in our culture largely because of our industrialized food system—a system that also includes unsustainable agricultural and environmental practices inconsistent with ecofeminist aims. The industrialized food system has alleviated human suffering on one hand and caused environmental damage on the other.

Carol Adams (1993) argues that animal rights will not permit tolerance of omnivorous food practices on cultural grounds. Many nutritionists do believe that vegans in "developing" countries have a poor health status attributable to "environmental factors (such as lack of medical care, vaccination, education and sanitation) rather than solely to diet" (Dwyer and Loew 1994, 88). That is, if we could improve background conditions to match those of the United States, then supplemented vegan diets would constitute little risk in the developing world. We might conclude that the risks would then be equalized (although burdens would not be equalized) among the sexes and ages, at least in theory. But, exporting safe vegan or vegetarian diets to the rest of the developing world requires exporting our food system with its fortification of cereals and other foods, processing of foods like egg substitutes, calcium-fortified soy products, and so forth. Fortification and food processing presuppose a complex industrialized food system, with research biochemistry, food processing plants, mines to produce supplements, quality control bureaucracies, food preservation techniques, refrigeration, shipping, and perhaps even chemical-dependent agriculture. All of these aspects of our food systems have environmental consequences, many or most of which are at odds with ecofeminist ideals. If one argues that these institutions should be reduced, eliminated, or radically altered as seems to be implied in Adams' and many other ecofeminist arguments, then a return to whole foods and unsupplemented or less supplemented diets is implied or may be a corollary. Eliminating or downscaling the industrialized food production process may mean that cereals and infant formulas may not be iron-fortified, milk may not have vitamin D added (if dairy is consumed), soy milk may not be calcium-fortified, and vitamin B_{12} may be unavailable for vegans. Very likely, human suffering would increase. Such circumstances would place even greater burdens on women, children, and others unless diet is adjusted to personal physiology and consumption of animal flesh and animal products continues in moderation. Deindustrialization of agriculture and the scientific food production process suggests that at least some animal agriculture and fishing should be maintained to assure that infants, children, adolescents, the elderly, pregnant and lactating women have good sources of iron, zinc, and vitamin B_{12} (meat/flesh of animals), calcium and B_{12} (dairy), vitamin D (eggs and fatty fish). And as I have said, even an industrialized food system places discriminatory burdens on these groups, despite mitigation by supplementation.[33]

Thus, any moral view that directs us to vegetarianism will be hard-pressed to escape domination and exploitation of the earth, nonindustrialized cultures, and even of the animals it seeks to spare. It is more likely to preserve class distinctions and hierarchy than to dissipate them. Nutritional education, medical care, and dietary supplements should, of course, be made available to those who want them. Agreeing to these facts and values does not, however, commit us to the ethical vegan ideal. It would, at most, commit us to improving conditions for all human and nonhuman animals depending on ecosystem impacts and cultural conditions.

In chapter 6 I continue the discussion of how the male norm makes effective implementation of moral equality for females difficult or impossible.

SUMMARY

Ethical vegetarians such as Singer, Regan, and Adams argue for a *universal* moral rule that aims eventually to realize the vegan ideal for everyone everywhere. But in that case, they must accept the assumptions that attend the vegetarian lifestyle—that our Western way of life is best and being an adult male in that culture is best. On the other hand, they cannot accept these assumptions and remain consistent in their moral beliefs. The argument for ethical vegetarianism is logically founded on an even more fundamental moral principle—the Principle of Equality. People whose bodies differ from our own should not be arbitrarily required to bear greater burdens than we do. Likewise, we cannot simply assume that our culture is *morally* better than those in less developed countries because their practices differ from ours. Having our way of life depends on an industrialized complex that has implications for culture and the environment and requires a vast expenditure of labor and resources—wealth. The ethical arguments serve the powerful by making them appear to be more morally virtuous simply because they have the material means to live a certain kind of life without health consequences. The less-well-off appear to be morally inferior simply because they don't have these means. The ethic in this case comes to endorse a view that "might makes right."

If we really mean to take seriously the claim of every person to choose his or her own way of life, we must validate the many *perspectives* from which humans solve problems. This does not mean that we must validate *all* solutions or points-of-view, since we should still condemn the policies of some groups to exert a destructive and oppressive influence on the lives and opportunities of others. But the argument for a vegan ideal simply *excuses* all other "less advanced" societies as morally deficient by circumstance or by ignorance of the best way to live. But I say that rather than "forgive" and excuse Mr. Alessandro or Rachel and her children, we should question the foundations of our ethical system. Why should we think that our culture—with its attitude of dominating and manipulating nature for patriarchal ends—is the only one capable of a moral relationship to food animals?

Before the discussion of whether a feminist ethic can support ethical vegetarianism, I review in the next chapter possible sources of bias in the nutritional studies cited here. In meeting the possible objections, I elaborate my argument from this chapter and give you additional reasons, both objective and subjective, for the validity of my arguments and the truth of my claims.

CHAPTER 5

BIAS, REASONING, AND SCIENTIFIC STUDIES

INTRODUCTION

Chapter 4 makes extensive use of nutritional information that is gathered from the scientific literature. But, the nutritional studies or the researchers who did them could be biased, my use of the studies biased or slanted, or my interpretation of them could be incorrect. Some nutritional findings are in dispute, and this may cast doubt on the use of the facts in my argument. In addition, my conclusions might be improperly drawn from the facts and ethical principles presented. In this chapter, I examine briefly the kinds of bias and mistakes of reasoning that might enter these studies. I also explain the strategies I used and that nutritional researchers use to minimize bias.

BIAS

In Research Studies

Bias can enter nutritional research in a number of ways. Studies could be poorly designed so that the researchers only find the results they are already looking for. The study population could be chosen from people who are not representative of the larger affected population. Or, the researchers could simply draw the wrong conclusions from their data. Flaws in design may negate the findings or may simply make the study less reliable. A more pervasive bias could predispose the researcher to see the world in gender-biased and racially biased ways. All of these problems could occur at once.

Taking the broadest question first, is all or most nutrition research tainted by a gender-biased or racially biased worldview? If not, why not? If so, does such bias mean that all conclusions drawn from scientific studies are unreliable—is there any nutritional knowledge from research science?

Donna Haraway, Sandra Harding, and a number of other feminists have argued forcefully that Western science is male-dominated and male-biased in a number of different ways and that such an orientation affects the reality of what science discovers. A detailed discussion of feminist philosophy of science will not be possible here, but one main criticism questions the basic structure of science. Feminists critics charge that the whole research enterprise reflects a masculinist attitude that is Cartesian in its dualism and a devaluation of the body and the physical world. Science was constructed and is controlled even today by mostly white males of middle or upper class economic means. So, the perspectives and values of women and people of color have been omitted from the structure of science. This kind of bias can enter scientific research on the levels of who will conduct the research, who will be studied, the problems to be studied, assessment of the adequacy of methods, and interpretation of data (Gruen and Gaard 1995; Keller 1982).

Is all or most of the nutritional research cited in support of my argument so gender-biased or racially biased as to be unreliable? Several reasons argue against such a conclusion. First, if all or almost all nutritional research is unreliable, then ethical vegetarians would have no generalizable scientific knowledge about the relative burdens, benefits, or risks of vegan and vegetarian diets. In other words, if vegetarians cannot trust the evidence that some groups are nutritionally vulnerable and require extra care, then neither can they trust the evidence that vegan diets are safe.[1] Second, even if most science were biased, many nutritional studies likely reflect a more feminist, feminine, or womanly approach. Two reasons support this second claim. Much of the research on *deficiencies* has been done by women upon women and children (see my reference list and the bibliographies of the nutritional reviews cited). And, most of these women researchers are senior scientists who have designed their own studies based on their own questions and concerns. They are responsible for assessing the methods and interpreting the data. By contrast, studies on the *benefits* of vegetarian diets (that is, reduction in mortality from coronary and ischemic heart disease, lower cancer rates, lower blood pressure) have largely been done on males by male scientists. As I said in chapter 4, the latter are unfairly biased if extrapolated to women, children, and others not fitting the male physiological norm.

The studies supporting my claims that the vegan ideal imposes an unequal burden on these people more closely reflect the concerns and thoughts of women and should be freer of objectionable bias.

Bias may remain in the hierarchy of science, but would that be sufficient to negate all of the findings about observed deficiencies in infants and gestating and lactating women? It would not. Although women studying women would not guarantee escape from a gender-biased Cartesian scientific paradigm, two more considerations argue for a reduction in such bias. First, feminists have argued that womanly ways of knowing and judging the world differ from the more typically masculine ways (for instance, Harding 1991; Alcoff and Potter 1993). These womanly scientists would be at least as unlikely to leave their unique interests and ways of knowing outside the lab as masculinist scientists would be in leaving their predominant worldview outside.

Second, one should distinguish a philosophy of science from the aims of scientific method in study design. To say that science is prey to a Cartesian dualism is to claim that it operates under a false philosophy of science. The bias thus introduced differs from what might be introduced by a faulty study design. Because of prevailing philosophical, cultural, social, political, and scientific paradigms, constructivist and feminist philosophies of science predict that all studies are likely to be biased in that the subjectivity of the researcher cannot be eliminated. But bias and subjectivity are not coextensive. Bias implies preference for a certain outcome or a tendency to see in a limited direction. Subjectivity acknowledges the particularity of point-of-view of individual consciousness. Having only one vantage point does not imply objectionable bias nor does it rule out having some knowledge. Some studies may be more subjective than others, and because science, like other institutions, is heavily male-dominated, the importance of looking for masculinist bias should remain a priority. But subjectivity alone does not preclude knowing. If it did, we should all embrace solipsism and desist from speaking and arguing.

The research conclusions could also be biased by one or more false presuppositions in all or most of the studies. Nutritionists might presuppose that vegetarian diets are deficient and then look for groups to study to "prove" it. Dwyer and Loew (1994) note that studies of lifelong Seventh-Day Adventist vegetarians in the 1950s and 1960s in the United States showed that these groups were generally healthy when they ate well-planned diets supplemented with some vitamins and minerals at appropriate times, had healthy habits, and received adequate medical care. In the 1970s, studies of "new" vegetarians were done. Because these groups adopted vegetarian diets as adults for religious or philosophical reasons, nutritionally vulnerable groups did not always fare as well.

"Lack of knowledge about nutrition, mistrust of the medical establishment, and limited access to foods considered acceptable led to deficiencies of energy . . . and of nutrients such as iron . . . , vitamin D . . . , and protein . . . , especially among children" (Mangels and Havala 1994, 112). Dwyer and Loew (1994) review the limitations of such studies, but argue that certain kinds of bias are not objectionable because of the good aims of researchers:

> Clinical nutrition is prevention- and treatment-oriented and thus it regards even small preventable risks as important, especially when the risks are serious. Also, health professionals believe that they have an ethical obligation and legal liability to alert patients about the potential adverse effects, however rare, of alternative dietary practices, including vegan diets, megadosing with vitamins and minerals, fad weight loss diets, atherogenic diets, and the like (99).

In the United States a large number of processed, pre-prepared, and fortified foods are available that make becoming a vegan far easier than it was only a few years ago—an accomplishment attributable to our industrialized and highly technological food system. Vitamin and mineral deficiencies such as pellagra were common in the United States at the turn of this century, but today are virtually nonexistent.[2] Nevertheless, cases of pellagra, beriberi, scurvy, megaloblastic anemia, iron deficiency anemias, and other dietary deficiencies in the First World are reported in the literature every year. In many places in the Third World, such deficiencies are endemic.[3]

Finally, most nutritionists agree that virtually every healthy person in the United States could adopt vegan diets with proper supplementation, education, and health care (Havala and Dwyer 1988, 1993; Dwyer and Loew 1994). So, it seems unlikely that these researchers or nutritionists are intentionally or unintentionally predisposed to study groups that would prove such diets unhealthy.

INTERPRETATION AND SLANT

Even if the nutrition literature is balanced, my argument depends upon presenting an "all-things-considered" or fair interpretation of the scientific conclusions. Both sides of a question should be presented if there is genuine dispute. For example, in defense of unsupplemented diets, vegans often tell me that plant foods contain as much calcium as milk and as much iron as meat, and claim that vegans, presumably of any age, can obtain adequate intakes from all-plant diets. For instance: "calorie for calorie, spinach, lettuce, green beans, tofu, and black-eyed peas all contain more iron than even the leanest cuts of sirloin steak"

(Varner 1994a, 34), and that "a portion" of such foods each contains similar amounts of iron (Pluhar 1993, 40). Are these statements correct? No, they are not. The statements are misleading because neither considers the bulk in most of these foods and their relatively low calorie content. First, heme (meat-source) iron is better absorbed than nonheme (plant-source) iron, but setting that aside for the moment, a fourteen-year-old girl would have to eat four cups of lettuce (0.8 mg Fe/cup), ¾ cup spinach (4 mg Fe/cup), or 2.5 cups of green beans (1.2 mg Fe/cup) to get the same 3 mg of iron (Fe) as in a 3-ounce lean hamburger patty (twenty-five percent of her RDA). The amount of energy (kcal) provided is not similar. From these "portions" the hamburger provides 190 kcal; the lettuce, 40 kcal; the spinach, 30 kcal; the green beans, 75 kcal (calculated from values in Saltman *et al.* 1987).[4] Teenagers are still growing and require more energy than adults. Infants and younger children are adding tissue continuously in growth and the stomach capacity of a young child is too small to permit digesting large amounts of fibrous foods; the low caloric content in these foods may not meet the energy needs of young children and may put them "at risk of inadequate intake of calories" (Jacobs and Dwyer 1988, 813).

What about the conclusions I report on calcium and osteoporosis? Lacto-vegetarians or lactoovovegetarians would be expected to have high calcium intakes, and indeed lifelong high milk intake is correlated with lower rates of osteoporosis (Barrett-Connor *et al.* 1994). So, the concern arises only for vegans. Long-term studies of vegan women and osteoporosis incidence have not been done. Still, moral vegans argue for removing milk from children's diets. The Physicians Committee for Responsible Medicine (PCRM) promotes vegan diets for everyone and aligns itself with the animal rights movement. PCRM claims that "green leafy vegetables such as kale are as good or better than milk as calcium sources" (quoted in Liebman 1992). Liebman (1992), writing for the Center for Science in the Public Interest, disputes this claim with known facts: "A cup of milk has 300 to 350 mg of calcium. A cup of cooked kale has 90 to 180 mg. And how many kids eat kale by the cup?" (2). Also, young children must have enough calories for growth, and milk provides a compact source of protein.[5] PCRM has no studies that kale will actually protect children from osteoporosis later in life, whereas studies in the United States and from less industrialized China (Hu *et al.*1993) have shown that women who report consuming more dairy products in adolescence have higher bone densities in later life than women who did not. The evidence is regarded as conclusive that milk protects, whereas the jury is yet to be formed on kale.[6]

Some moral vegans claim that it would be safer for infants and children to avoid nonhuman milk because cow's milk is not needed for health (PCRM

1991) and can cause allergies (Pluhar 1992). Soy-based formulas can be substituted when breast milk is absent. Here, the bias and slant occur in their claims, not mine. Some infants do exhibit allergies to cow's milk, but that does not mean cow's milk is unsafe in general. Every choice involves some risks, and some infants have exhibited allergies to soy-based formulas as well (Bardare *et al.* 1988; Sorensen *et al.* 1993); "it has been shown that legumes (soy) occupy the fourth place in importance among the food allergens, inducing hypersensitivity reactions in Spanish children" (Carrillo Díaz 1986, 145). Olejer (1993) lists peanuts and soy along with milk and eggs as accounting for "eighty percent to ninety percent of the food allergy reactions diagnosed in the first few years of life. . . . There is no universally safe food" (212).

Parents must decide what is best for their children on balance, given family history, economic considerations, and physician's recommendations. Having a variety of nutritional sources assures that virtually every child will have an alternative in case of contraindication or allergic response to a particular food. Moreover, because we know that moral commitments take precedence over perceived personal self-interest, a parent's commitment to the vegan ideal may have the effect of blocking acceptance of proper nutrition, even if dairy products or another essential nutrient source were needed to provide it.[7]

Although bias and poor study design do appear in some individual published studies, it does not follow that the major conclusions of all the research taken together are wrong. Reviews and studies should be evaluated on their own merits. The best way to avoid being swayed by bias is to read widely and attempt to understand with an open mind. The findings reported here reflect corroboration, not from a few studies here or there, but from cumulative evidence of thousands and thousands of studies done by researchers from all sorts of laboratories, most of which are in university rather than corporate or governmental settings.

REDUCING SOME TYPES OF BIAS

How can a person tell which studies to trust? One criterion calls for examining the internal aspects of study design. The primary aims of study design are to rule out objectionable bias as far as possible and to discover causal relationships among events in the world. Some designs yield better reliability than others (Giere 1991; see also Dwyer and Loew 1994 for review of how bias can enter research on vegan and vegetarian populations). Their relative reliability, from most to least, is as follows: (1) double-blind[8] trials; (2) blind trials; (3) prospective studies; and (4) retrospective studies.[9] All good studies should include a control group. The first three types also use randomized processes to select and assign subjects to the experimental or control groups. Subjects are randomly selected to try to assure that the researcher is not getting a group that exhibits the phenomenon in question more often than the whole affected population would. If an hypothesis has been tested and confirmed in study after study, then a real causal relationship is highly probable, even if a few experiments do not confirm the hypothesis (see Giere 1991 and Copi and Cohen 1990). In human clinical testing, ethical considerations often preclude doing the most reliable types of studies (Royall 1991). So, prospective and retrospective studies are used, and many more corroborative reports and large samples are need to increase the reliability of the results.

In their reports, scientists always review similar studies because an hypothesis can only be tested in context. Review reports can be a good place for nonscientists to look for a summary of the most current evidence about any particular problem. However, every scientific discipline relies on specialized testing procedures, each of which has its own relative reliability. For instance, nutrition studies rely on excretion studies of specific minerals such as calcium (in urine) and iron (in blood loss); reports of daily food intakes over a specific time period; the use of radiography, spectroscopy, and other instruments which measure the uptake of vitamins and minerals into the body, and many other procedures, all offering different confidence levels for belief. Attempting to analyze the meaning of particular studies requires a thorough acquaintance with the methodological pitfalls of testing procedures in a particular study area and an understanding of the historical context.[10]

The news media often report correlations and single studies, but innumerable events occur together, some of which are co-incidental and some of which are causally related (see Liebman 1994 for a well-written synopsis of how to judge nutrition research results). Correlations must be analyzed and tested to see whether their occurrence together is significantly greater than what could be expected by chance. Even in causal relations, interactions and intervening steps may mask determining causes.[11] For moral arguments, a person must know the facts before she can take the right action. She must be able to say with reasonable certainty, for instance, that lack of vitamin B_{12} *causes* (or does not cause) megaloblastic anemia.[12] Requiring people to take moral action on the basis of sheer speculation, simple correlation, anecdotal reports, poorly constructed studies, one or two disconfirming reports in the face of other substantial confirmation, or hypothesis alone would often require them to do contradictory and even harmful actions since many hypotheses, correlations, and anecdotes give reasons to perform conflicting actions. Some past examples of actions based on false correlations include witch-burning and using "snake oil."

Paying attention to study design does not guarantee a value-free, bias-free study, but the design is intended to reduce bias. When scientific evidence conflicts, as it often does, readers should study the conflicting reports for racial and gender bias, the reliability of the methods used, the construction of the experimental group, the presence of confounding factors, the likelihood of the results occurring by chance (whether results are significant), check statistical analyses for accuracy, and so forth. Reading widely and in depth is the best way to assure yourself that you are getting the best all-things-considered opinions.

DISPUTES IN NUTRITION RESEARCH

Anyone who consults the scientific literature in nutrition will find that disagreements exist about some facts such as necessary levels and sources for certain requirements; for example, calcium. But the presence of disagreement does not negate the more general claims. My argument does not depend on questions at the edge of present knowledge in nutrition. Some questions are the basis for ongoing research, and at the edge of knowledge there are no noncontroversial answers. Disputes are the grist of inquiry in science and in ethics as well. But inquiry is made possible because some facts are not in dispute and are well-corroborated. For example: calcium is required for skeletal growth and maintenance; bone loss occurs gradually after age thirty; women have smaller skeletons than men; women of Japanese and European descent have, on average, smaller skeletons than women of African descent and are thus more predisposed to osteoporosis; calcium supplementation and milk consumption do prevent acceleration of bone loss and osteoporosis. The preponderance of current controversy centers on how much supplementation and dietary source calcium should be recommended *above* the RDA, because the RDAs are constantly being revised in light of new knowledge. Similarly, scientists have shown beyond question the importance of iron to pregnant women and infants; in large part that is the justification for fortifying cereals, soy milk, and infant formulas with iron.[13]

PERSONAL BIAS AND PERSONAL ENLIGHTENMENT

As I have said above, no one can completely eliminate her own subjectivity from any research project and I am no exception. But knowledge is still possible, and some strategies exist for limiting objectionable kinds of bias. Perhaps if I had some vested interest in the food animal industry, that would limit my ability to present the best "all-things-considered" information about the nutritional differentials among women, children, the old, and adult men. But I am a philosophy professor who was already a vegetarian at the beginning of my quest. I came to the research as woman academically trained in biology and in traditional moral theory, won over to an ethical vegetarian position by Tom Regan's arguments. I am also a mother, a wife, a food preparer, and a feminist. What should I expect my daughter to eat? What should I prepare for her? Those contexts and questions were and are at the center of my subjectivity. I am semivegetarian today, but I believe that is not generalizable in a moral principle, not idealizable in matters of virtue, and feminist in its formulation.

I didn't come to that conclusion when I first read the nutrition literature. I learned almost immediately that vegan women in the United States and Europe apparently have no difficulty maintaining the RDAs if they are careful to eat a balanced diet and take supplements where needed. Many of our foods are already fortified with vitamins and minerals, making it seem as if our diet "naturally" contains everything we need for health. At first I thought that, because women, children, and older people can take supplements and eat fortified foods to make up for what their vegan diets may lack, morality still required them all to be vegetarians at least and maybe even vegans. I considered removing the dairy products and shellfish from my diet, but I still had not decided what to teach my daughter and whether to encourage her to restrict her diet at all. I wondered whether my (by then) eleven-year-old daughter would realize her full health potential without milk or meat—would she be more vulnerable to osteoporosis in older age or to iron deficiency anemia and its side-effects in adolescence and later (assuming she continued the diet after she leaves home)? In other words, would I be harming her eventually by imposing a diet upon her based on my well-intentioned moral beliefs? Since I was perimenopausal, I wondered whether I would risk accelerated bone loss and eventual osteoporosis without dairy products. Even that might constitute a harm to her if it fell to her to care for me in a frail condition.

Adult men didn't seem to have these worries. It didn't seem fair that I or my children should have to live as men were better suited to live. The *burden* for us is greater, even if the risks can be equalized. Earlier in my life I had worked with low-income people who were ill. I realized that buying vitamins and supplements and even some types of healthy foods is a much greater economic burden for them than for a middle-income or wealthy person. It didn't seem fair to require them to be vegans or to idealize that lifestyle and then grant them a "hardship excuse." But the vegan life still appeared to be the highest life. Vegans were still somehow better people, or at least they appeared to be if their moral ideas were correct.[14] It struck me that it was a whole lot easier for adult men to be "better people" than it was for me and my daughter. Ordinarily, they didn't have to worry at all about iron deficiency anemia, and any concerns they might have about osteoporosis would crop up only if they lived into their late eighties or nineties.

Removing meat from my diet at my age in 1986 really caused me no particular health burden nor did I find it any particular culinary hardship. I've always preferred vegetables. I could expect my iron status to remain stable because I was using birth control pills (which reduce blood loss at menstruation) and I planned to have no more children. But then I began to think beyond my own age and reproductive status. Like Penny in chapter 1 and many other pregnant women, twelve years earlier I had anemia severe enough to be advised to have a blood transfusion (partially secondary to continuous spotting) despite taking an iron supplement and eating lots of dark green vegetables. My obstetrician suggested that I eat beef liver several times a week to increase the absorption of iron and I did.[15] If moral vegetarianism were required, I would have been entitled to an exemption from the vegan ideal based on what Regan calls the Liberty Principle. My anemia abated. Comparing that time to my position in 1986, I realized that simply by growing older and barren, I seem to have become better—more virtuous. Whereas in 1976 I was an omnivore with an excuse, now I could be an ideal vegetarian and maybe even a vegan. Now I knew something was wrong with the whole argument. We may get wiser simply from getting older and more experienced, but virtue is not a function of age or body type. Virtue or personal goodness is a function of a moral character shaped by individual choice. But how does a pregnant woman have a choice to live as a virtuous vegan in the face of anemia? She has to hope that the "defect" (of being pregnant) will pass so that she, too, may hope to attain the epitome of goodness.

It is, of course, possible that these experiences have created an objectionable bias in my argument. I leave it to you to expose such flaws. I do agree that the experience was valuable in that it helped me to uncover the contradictions in ethical vegetarian arguments.

MISTAKES OF REASONING

FACTS AND VALUES

In ethics, people sometimes try to draw moral conclusions from facts alone, thereby committing the "is-ought" fallacy.[16] The fallacy involves an *enthymeme*, or elliptical argument. That is, one or more of the premises of the argument are unspoken, assumed, or unstated. Nevertheless, the premise is still recoverable by reflecting on the conclusion. For instance, my daughter may point out the facts:

"You promised to take me to the next volleyball game. The next game is tomorrow." From that she may plausibly draw the moral conclusion: "You should take me to the game tomorrow." The argument is not necessarily fallacious, although she draws an "ought" from an "is." Implicit in her argument is the unstated moral assumption: "Promises ought to be kept." If the moral premise is assented to, then the argument is still valid. The fallacy arises from trying to get someone to assent to a moral conclusion by hiding a shaky moral premise.

If my argument in the previous chapter depended on drawing ethical conclusions from facts and an unstated moral premise, then my reasoning might be specious. But as you recall, the moral premises are explicitly stated—that discrimination based on being female, or young, or old is wrongful, that equity and impartiality are essential to traditionalist views of morality, and that affirmation of the female body is essential to feminist morality. These moral assumptions are defensible on independent grounds but are assumed only as essential to traditional and feminist formulations of ethics.

Nevertheless, the place of facts in moral arguments may still be questioned. In a post-positivist and post-Cartesian worldview, the demarcation between "is" and "ought" is necessarily blurred. The designation of "fact" cannot be value-free. Everything we believe stands or falls *within* a context, and no one can rise (or fall?) to a standpoint completely outside of human culture. The so-called facts are infected with "oughts," making it difficult to assess their relevance. Even so, some of our beliefs are more reliable than others, and referencing these in a moral argument is essential. Knowing these well-corroborated facts gives an understanding of the causes and consequences of what we do. Our actions may benefit or harm others. Because harms and unequal burdens are morally important in any ethical framework, then referencing them in support of our choices will be obligatory. If facts had no place in our moral argumentation, then all moral thinking would rely solely on mystical or charismatic declarations of faith. Notice that the ethical vegetarian relies on factual claims to say that these diets are safe and pose little or no risk. I simply claim that they still pose unequal burdens. If I am denied reference to facts, then so will they be. But then, ethical vegetarians must be willing to say their actions are right *no matter what the facts and no matter what the harms.*

Showing that ethical vegetarians have the facts wrong about the physiological interchangeability of human bodies does not, by itself, imply what anyone should do about being or remaining a vegetarian (or anything else for that matter). Values may stand while facts fall. That is why it is possible for someone to hold a self-sacrificial pacifism, a doctrine of human sacrifice or of white racial supremacy. The issue is whether, in the face of certain facts, we should continue to affirm certain values in an unaltered way. Because the nutritional claims that underlie traditional moral arguments are mistaken, the primary support for ethical vegetarianism is removed. Facts act as the reasons one has to hold a particular belief. If there are now no good reasons to hold a belief, then it is apparently arbitrary. One must either find new reasons—which could be new facts or other values—or one must give up the belief. So, at the very least, a full understanding of the facts about unsupplemented vegetarian diets and human physiology undermines support for the traditional and feminist arguments for ethical vegetarianism.

Additionally, it is not as if new knowledge has suddenly come to light that women and children are nutritionally vulnerable. That has been known for decades. As in other cases of discrimination, important facts were overlooked or downplayed in order to make the kind of argument traditional moralists and some feminists wished to make. Nor have our values changed—women and children *are* as intrinsically important as men. Reminding traditional moralists of the relevant differences between age groups, sexes, classes, and cultures does make the question of fair treatment of nonhuman animals more complex, but it does not present new values.

Indigenous Knowledge versus Scientific Knowledge

So far, I have relied heavily on scientifically trained nutritionists for validation of the fact that certain groups are nutritionally vulnerable and face greater burdens on vegetarian diets. Yet, food preparers, usually women, often have a great store of cultural knowledge of food and nutrition gained without science. Traditional recipes often combine local foods in ways that balance nutrients, and women gatherers use indigenous food sources unknown to the grocery store set. Such knowledge is being rapidly lost in "developing" nations with the advance of industrialized, unsustainable farming methods and food distribution systems. Despite my reliance on empirical science, everything I have said supports prizing such indigenous knowledge, preserving it, and learning from it. Nutritional anthropologists often seek to learn about that knowledge by living in a household and observing the patterns of food acquisition, exchange, recipe making, food preparation and distribution (Sharman *et al.* 1991). Although they have found so far that families have many ways of supplying required nutrients and coping with food shortages, no indication has arisen that women and children in these cultures are physiologically *less nutritionally vulnerable* on unsupplemented vegan or vegetarian diets. No amount of indigenous knowledge can make up for the fact that there are no plant sources of vitamin B_{12}, for instance. History shows that it is simply false that traditional diets in "obligatory vegan cultures" are largely healthful or that nutritional deficiencies in women and children are caused only by food shortages and power structures. Even in areas of the world where food is in sufficient supply and is least disrupted by modern agriculture, nutritional deficiencies remain (pellagra in Indonesia, beriberi, iron deficiency and rickets in India, deficiencies in China).

Americans should not underestimate the power of their ideals to profoundly affect the course of other cultures. The vegan ideal may actually be contributing to the loss of indigenous nutritional knowledge—knowledge that will be better preserved if it is not judged by an ideal morality condemning all animal production. For instance, food shortages and nutritional deficiencies are endemic to certain parts of the world (Scrimshaw 1990). In these areas, Americans have often engaged in public or private (tax-funded or charitable) efforts to provide humanitarian aid. While well-intentioned, food aid and farming aid have both hastened the loss of indigenous knowledge (Lappé and Collins 1986; Norgaard 1987; Shiva 1989, 1991) by (among other things) disrupting land use and local growing and gathering patterns, and destroying indigenous species as well as by dislocating families and communities from each other and their regions of origin.

PERSPECTIVE AND THE AIMS OF ETHICS

So I wondered, from whose perspective shall we decide whether vegetarianism is morally required? From the perspective of largely white, relatively affluent adult Western males? Or from the perspective of Third World women or their children? Shall we ask these questions from the perspective of the powerful or the vulnerable? Yes, in the United States we can take supplements. But, that fact does not address my charges of ageism, sexism, or cultural bias. For even if it is not too risky for a middle-class infant, child, adolescent, pregnant, lactating, perimenopausal, post-menopausal, or elderly female to be a vegan or vegetarian in the United States that judgment will surely be made from a male-biased perspective of assuming that all those women, children, and seniors can fix, mend, or correct their imperfect bodies as necessary (by supplementation, fortified foods, or eating in special ways) to meet a vegan ideal that is much less burdensome for men. Simply because risk may be equalized does not mean that burdens are equalized. If the adult wealthy male is not the paradigm, then the benchmark for the assessment of risk will be different. If women's bodies, or children's bodies, are benchmarks instead, then different kinds of assumptions will be made, and these will affect how we think about our bodies and our food.

The answer also depends on a certain view of the aims of ethics. If you believe that the ethical codes and beliefs of a society are there and *should be there* to protect the rich and the powerful, their rights and privileges, then perhaps you will *not* agree with these arguments. But I believe that ethics should consider the welfare of the vulnerable and not just the powerful. So, some attempt must be made to draft an ethics which accounts for and concerns itself with the perspectives of the very differently situated people and animals with whom we share the earth. Only in that way will ethics truly be for everyone. As I argue in chapter 6, a feminist ethic will take account of equality and difference, and in chapter 7 I show that the most consistent feminist position on diet is a feminist aesthetic semivegetarianism.

CHAPTER 6

GENDER EQUALITY AND INTERSPECIES EQUALITY

———————————————

DO PHYSIOLOGICAL DIFFERENCES REQUIRE INEQUALITY?

In chapter 4, the nutritional information illuminates some of the possible contexts where women, children, and others may find themselves on unequal footing if they were to adopt moral vegetarianism. These contexts of inequality are many and varied. They are ever-changing within a single life that stretches from birth, infancy, adolescence, child-bearing, menopause, and old age. Supplementation may alleviate physiological risks for women, children, and others, but increases their burdens. Ethical vegetarianism presupposes a health ideal rooted in the positive reality of the adult male body and the inherent lack of the bodies of the others to measure up to that norm.[1] Likewise, the superiority of First World culture and ways of life is assumed. But, as I have said from the beginning, no feminist ethics can tolerate an ethical approach based on such claims.

While some feminists, such as Carol Adams, apparently base their ethical vegetarianism on traditional moral theory, many others reject or attempt to modify traditional rights and utilitarian approaches.[2] In chapter 3, I gave a brief summary of some feminist approaches to ethical vegetarianism, including some that attempt to begin from other than traditionalist ground. In this chapter, I return to the question of whether some version of a feminist ethic could support vegetarianism *as a condition of being moral.* Keep in mind that, given access to supplements and fortified foods, vegetarianism is not a bad practice. It is not unethical or wrongful, even for groups whose risks and burdens are higher. This text is about whether vegetarianism is *required* for most ordinary people. Feminists may adopt vegetarianism. I am merely arguing that people should not idealize the vegan life nor urge it upon others in the belief that the practice is necessary to being truly ethical, to being a consistent feminist or ecofeminist, or to live by the principle of equality. Quite the contrary. It is *impossible* to honor equality and claim that equality demands ethical vegetarianism.

THE MINIMUM CONCEPTION OF FEMINIST ETHICS

When I began this book, I stated that anyone committed to two basic beliefs that I call the "minimum conception of a feminist ethics" must reject ethical vegetarianism. These two beliefs are: First, no ethics can admit of arbitrariness in its prescriptions and theories. Second, any specifically feminist ethic must affirm the value of the female body. Whatever else a feminist ethics is or will be, it must reject requiring women to live as if physiologically identical to men and assigning arbitrary moral burdens and/or benefits to women or other persons based on factors that cannot be changed by human choice. On the basis of the evidence in chapter 4, the nutritional contexts already show that these two assumptions have been violated by most versions of feminist ethical vegetarianism because an adult male norm is assumed.

Even though the nutrition literature has for decades reported the empirical differences in dietary requirements at different stages of life and across sexes (as reflected in the RDAs, for instance), those arguing for the vegan ideal probably did not notice that they were basing their arguments on a false premise—that we are all the same. Traditional philosophers are used to thinking in terms of the equality of persons. Each person is to be accorded equal respect and equal treatment. We are supposed to disregard certain kinds of differences between us and pay attention to the sameness among us. Many of the differences we are to disregard concern the appearance and function of the body, such as skin color, racial characteristics, and gender. In hiring for a job, admitting a person to a program of study, or treating a person for an illness, it is wrong to consider the race or gender of a person. Recently, though, some feminists have pointed out that gender does make people differently situated. So, it is not always obvious when someone should take into account or disregard a particular difference or set of differences.

Recent applications of the principle of equality using traditional moral and legal theory have proven to be quite problematic. For example, scholarship in feminist legal theory points to many inconsistencies in judicial decisions concerning women in the work force (see Smith 1993). The writings of feminist legal scholars hold promise for developing an alternative view of feminist morality. In this chapter I suggest that their prescriptions for dealing with gender differences can be appropriately applied to the problem of species differences. I critically review feminist concerns about gender differences and equal treatment, and then I show how these arguments may be applied to species equality. In chapter 7, I reconsider "contextual moral vegetarianism" primarily from the view of Deane Curtin, and I explain why this view will not support feminist ethical vegetarianism. Finally, I endorse a feminist aesthetic semivegetarianism as most consistent with feminism.

EQUALITY AND DIFFERENCE

EQUALITY AND SAMENESS

First-wave feminists used the language of rights, justice, and equality to gain suffrage and opportunities in public life (Wollstonecraft 1792, Mill 1869). These feminists argued that women and men are materially the same in their ability to reason and to learn. Because both sexes have the same capacities, both should be recognized as morally equal and given similar liberties and opportunities. Although these appeals were eventually effective, many feminists today question whether the liberal tradition and its view of the self and equality can be reformed to accommodate important *differences* of gender, sexual orientation, race, handicap, culture, and ethnicity. The scholarship of many feminists led to the realization that women, in virtue of their unique capacity for menstruation, child-bearing, lactation, and menopause are quite differently situated than are men. Because of these capacities women experience the world differently. We are not the *same*. That males and females are not materially identical or interchangeable seems obvious. It's just that the differing characteristics between them were deemed morally unimportant for implementing equality. The general political position of women as subordinates or as oppressed also makes women differently situated socially. Women of color and people from nonwestern cultures are likewise differently situated. In fact, all those not of a privileged class experience life and society in ways the dominant class cannot. Even as the language of rights affirms moral equality, that language abstracts away the crucial personal features of one's life, such as age, race, gender, sexual orientation, ethnicity and class. Such a notion of justice cannot consider the fact that some members of the moral community are neither autonomous nor materially equal and that partiality for members of one's family has ethical value.

Compounding the difficulty, traditional moral theory incorporates the apposition of dualistic categories such as masculine/feminine, reason/emotion, objective/subjective that reinforce role stereotypes and prejudices. These dualisms obscure the reality of the "same" and the "different" by evaluating one side of a dichotomy as "good" and the other as "bad." Why does this happen? Western moral thought usually posits a *common human nature* that is or can be shared by all. Some people live in accordance with their nature and others go against it. The former are good, the latter are bad—"saints and sinners," so to speak. Unfortunately, our moralistic thinking has tended to align male/female, reason/emotion, good/bad vertically, as in male/reason/good and female/emotion/bad. Thus, whatever is stereotypically associated with "masculine" has met with approbation while the "feminine" has met with opprobrium. And today, many, if not most, philosophers and feminists point out that criteria for a common human nature or essence of humanity are nonexistent.

A debate has ensued among feminists about the benefits and dangers of emphasizing women's differences from men. The primary danger is that it affirms feminine "essentialism" and offers superficial credence to the conservative view that women's intrinsic differences make them "naturally" suited to their traditionally subordinate place in society. Yet, as Patricia Smith comments, "this view is antithetical to any feminist position and should not be confused with the difference side of the feminist debate. All feminists hold that women are first and foremost human beings who are entitled to choose their own future from the full range of choices available to all human beings" (1993, 23). Equality requires fair treatment that accommodates both material similarities and differences. This means that *moral equality* cannot be founded solely upon *material equality*, as the liberal tradition had once assumed.

Gender Equality: Assimilation

Revisioning the principle of equality has been of particular concern to writers in feminist jurisprudence. Much of their writing has been a response to the *assimilation model* of equality: to be treated the same as men, women should live up to the same expectations as proposed for their male counterparts. Thus, they would be "assimilated" to the male ideal. The assimilation model becomes particularly problematic in areas where women are differently situated from men. Concrete cases involving pregnancy, childbirth, fetal endangerment, childcare, and other "family issues" have helped to illuminate the various ways in which law and precedent have presupposed male norms and the law's preference for a male physiology and masculine social situation. Herma Hill Kay

(1985) discusses several state court decisions on pregnancy and maternity leave as well as the Supreme Court decision that exclusion of pregnancy benefits from medical insurance plans is constitutional and that such benefits are not guaranteed by the equal protection clause: "The Court's false conclusion was that pregnant persons are not women. That conclusion led to the improper legal result that women were protected against sex discrimination only when they are like men—that is, when they are not pregnant" (43). Such court decisions have been "useless or detrimental to women because [they] are based on an initial requirement of material equality to men" (Smith 1993, 21).[3] That the Court permitted individual women *who measure up to the expectations of a male* to be treated the same as men illustrates the expectation that women should be "assimilated" to the male ideal.

Although equality does require that differences such as the capacity for pregnancy be accommodated, the Court focused on identifying like cases based on relevant material similarities and then deciding how to treat these cases alike. If people are different but still equal, the Court decided it had nothing to say. Patricia Smith (1993) points out, though, that the traditional principle of equality directs that different cases should be treated in proportion to their differences. Precious little work has been done to elucidate the meaning of that aspect of the principle. Nevertheless, law and morality have always recognized that people are often materially and socially *unequal.* "The presumption of equality . . . did not mean that all men were to be treated equally. Instead, it meant that unequal treatment had to be justified. That is, it did not deny inequality altogether; it merely shifted the burden of proof" (Smith 1993, 18).

Some feminists initially accepted the assimilation model and argued for "special rights" for women (for instance, Wolgast 1980). More recently, feminists have proposed reconceptualizing the norm or resolving the issue by setting aside concerns about equality and difference in favor of more pressing concerns about power and domination (see Taub and Williams 1985, Scales 1986, Littleton 1987, MacKinnon 1989; all reprinted in Smith 1993).

GENDER EQUALITY: EMPOWERMENT

In an attempt to hurdle the same/difference dilemma, Ann Scales (1986) argues for an *empowerment model.* Following Catherine MacKinnon (1979), she argues that "law must embrace a version of equality that focuses on the real issues—domination, disadvantage and disempowerment—instead of on the interminable and diseased issue of differences between the sexes" (101). MacKinnon even calls her view the "inequality approach." Scales and MacKinnon are concerned that the law should protect women from "systematic subordination because of sex." Scales recognizes that, in deciding what constitutes domination and disadvantage, judges have traditionally relied on some "objective" notion of similarity and difference. But she is concerned that power should not be apportioned on the basis of a version of objectivity and equality that presupposes a male paradigm. Because differences are deep and real, attempts to establish one normatively objective standard of reference will fail and will be unjust.

Before I examine the applicability of the empowerment model to arguments for the equality of animals, a few general comments are in order. I admire the empowerment approach, but I think it begs the question. First, the concepts that Scales and MacKinnon recommend to our attention—domination, disadvantage, disempowerment—have become increasingly pejorative terms for at least two centuries as the circle of equality has expanded. Domination has not always been regarded as wrong. These conditions are thought to be unjust now simply because we have come to value equality. The full implementation of equality would at least minimize the occurrence of domination, disadvantage, and disempowerment in human relations. So, the argument assumes we already know what equality is. In order to understand what kinds of situations and experiences involve domination, disadvantage, and disempowerment, one must already know what it is to be entitled to a greater degree of power and advantage than one has and *why one is entitled to it.* No matter what wealth, power, and position people may have, without a framework for understanding the fair distribution of these goods, disputes over who is being dominated and disempowered dissolve into a cacophony of angry assertions sometimes followed by violence. MacKinnon (1989) seems quite willing to acknowledge the political nature of her claims. But people's perceptions of when they are being dominated or disempowered vary immensely and may be unreasonable and unfair. Legitimate conflicts of interest exist among humans—the best jobs have more qualified applicants than can be accommodated—no matter whether the reward is money or personal fulfillment. Some method, other than appeal to pure power, for adjudicating claims among moral equals who are materially unequal needs to be in place in order to end domination and disadvantage.

Second, Christine Littleton (1987) also points out that the empowerment model does not escape the male norm. The notion of power is that of "male-power" and social institutions that purport to be gender neutral are phallocentric. Thus, "empowering women without dealing with difference, like assimilation, too easily becomes simply sharing male power more broadly" (117). But, the empowerment model may be limited to the framework of constitutional law. Jurists are attempting practical implementations of a not-very-well-defined ideal.

Third, Scales notes that focusing on differences, such as exist in reproductive capacities between the sexes, denies us the kind of abstract objectivity needed for legal (and moral) judgment. No androgyne exists, nor would we want one. I interpret her to mean that because a purely *human* norm cannot be conceptualized, then we must circumvent thinking about dual norms. Some differences are incommensurable and make assessments of similarity impossible. Scales' tack is to "think about something else." But why must there be a single human norm? Although issues become more complex, one can admit that the range of goods for human beings varies with gender, age, sexual preference, physical and mental capacities, culture, etc., and still say that judgments relying on some version of equality are possible.

GENDER EQUALITY: ACCEPTANCE

Christine Littleton (1987) reviews several proposed solutions to the sameness/difference debate. While she recognizes that "'equality' . . . can no longer be embraced unambivalently by feminists," she defends a "reconstruction of sexual equality" that she calls the *acceptance model* (111). In her view, the cultural and biological differences among women and men "must be equally valid and valuable" (114). Differences have been used to justify unequal treatment, and her model focuses on trying to eliminate the "unequal consequences of sex difference" rather than debating whether such differences are "real" or whether cultural differences are caused by biology: "It is the consequences of gendered difference, and not its sources, that equal acceptance addresses" (114). Her view is pragmatic: Think about what equality is *for* rather than what it *is*. She claims that equality is meant to assure that (presumably harmless) differences in lifestyle are *costless*. That is, no one is penalized by social institutions for choosing a female lifestyle or a male one. Rather than attempting to determine whether disadvantage is merely perceived or is real, Littleton takes the more pragmatic approach of asking legal justice to remove barriers and remedy situations where women and men have unequal opportunities. Her model avoids assimilation and accommodation because she recognizes that the norms assumed in the present social system are male-defined:

> The form of male power that constructs male dominance as a social
> system . . . can be viewed as concentrated in the hands of a few men
> who are at or near the top of intersecting hierarchies of sex, race,
> and class, reserved to those in what I will call the *club*. The consti-
> tutive form of male power exercised by the club is the power to set
> the terms by which all forms of human activity are given social

> meaning and social value. The power to define what is and is not a right, a legal interest, equality, justice, or law itself is power that constitutes a system. *It is the power to construct reality itself; it is the power to "speak the world"* (123, emphasis added).

By speaking to the *function* of equality rather than to its abstract content, Littleton is able to avoid the conundrum of how to base moral equality on material inequality. She also views the law itself as having the function of apportioning power, although she does not endorse its present operation. Women and men, after all, assess power in different ways: masculine power is power over others—dominance; feminine power is the capacity to help others—nurturance. Women who are admitted to power under the present system must "either speak in a male voice or remain silent. And since speech as it is used by the club is the power to silence others, we must agree to use our voices to silence other women" (124–25). The club will not tolerate our voices; entry requires that all enter transformed as "socially male, white, and upwardly mobile" (125).

In order to "rescue equality and destroy the club," Littleton proposes a stepwise process that reduces present inequalities across differences in context after context. Her approach is open to critique on "theoretical grounds," of course, because it deliberately lacks planning or any structured approach to rationalize it. But that is its strength rather than its weakness, at least from this feminist's point of view. Littleton can also retort that a requirement for a "structured" approach would always assume a male-dominance structure that tends to silence women. The stepwise approach should eventually reveal itself to have its own structure that will be evident in hindsight, just as the rationalization of the male dominance club is visible to us now in studying the cases, laws, and social institutions that once validated it.

Littleton proposes a "disparate impact doctrine" for use in slowly changing employment conditions and social institutions so that the impact of such differences as pregnancy are costless or at least cost less. Her aim is to effect an evolution rather than a revolution. While ambitious in its ultimate aims, her proposed methodology is modest and sound. It has precedence in the method of scientific discovery, where experimenters continually modify and reconceptualize the reality they are attempting to know and construct by comparing context after context laboriously to each other until understanding becomes more complete. She does not assume that she knows what equality is or will be, but only that it should be realizable and should function to permit the fullest possible realization of good outcomes for all. If properly applied, perhaps her doctrine could be applied to the differing needs of women and men, children and the aged with respect to diet.

Next, I consider in more detail whether moral equality can be applied or realized across species. Is one of these models appropriate for effecting species equality? If so, which one and would ethical vegetarianism be an appropriate aim? If none will apply, why not?

INTERSPECIES EQUALITY

EQUALITY AND SAMENESS

Because feminists have not extended the equality/difference debate to interspecies ethics, most, if not all, current arguments for feminist vegetarianism rely on a traditional exposition of the principle of equality for their force. Traditional moral arguments for ethical vegetarianism (such as those of Regan and Singer) rely on the material equality of animals and humans; that is, some version of essentialism or some "common animal nature" that makes humans and animals the same. Singer (1975, 1990) argues against speciesism as being the same kind of wrong as racism or sexism—"all animals are equal." In such arguments, an "animal norm" is posited that functions in place of the male norm in traditional morality. The criteria for identifying the equal worth of animals are capacities for experiencing suffering and death (or interest in not experiencing them). All *differences* across species are argued to be morally irrelevant, that is, unimportant. Every argument, whether traditionalist or feminist, upholding the rights, welfare, or good of animals and the correlate of ethical vegetarianism cites these criteria as the primary reasons in support of it (see Adams 1993, Collard 1989, Donovan 1990, Gaard 1993, Gruen 1993, Gruzalski 1983, Regan 1983, Singer 1975, 1990). But, the differences make all the difference to a cat *qua* cat. The differences rather than the similarities make the cat situated as a cat and not, say, as a rat. If the genders are differently situated and these differences are morally important, then surely the species are differently situated and such differences matter.

But attempts to treat men, women, children, and animals equally based on similarities result in discrimination towards most of the world's humans and domestic animals. Several tacks have been taken by the debaters on the question of the moral status of animals. The first and most common is to deny that equality applies to animals: "equality for humans, lesser status for animals." In this, the debaters talk past one another, each offering different criteria for deciding that animals and humans are materially "the same" or not the same. An example is the Regan-Frey debate about whether animals count or not. Although their books on the subject were published in the early 1980s, they still appear together and debate the topic at symposia in the same way.[4] The moral theory used by traditionalist interlocutors does not affect this debate. McCloskey (1979) and Regan (1983) each employ rights theory but come to opposite conclusions about whether animals have the same rights as humans because the decision about whether all animals are equal precedes theory deployment. Similarly, Frey (1983) and Singer (1975) both employ utilitarianism with opposing results. They are not arguing moral theory; they are arguing about the principle of equality. From chapter 3, you can see that feminists avoid ontological analysis to include animals in the moral realm. In an attempt at avoiding the essentialism that Regan and Singer embrace, thinkers like Donovan and Kheel appeal to our emotive understanding of the pain and suffering of animals. I have argued that while we do have moral obligations to animals, agreeing about their equality in the face of obligations to family members and other people is much more problematic. As I have argued in previous chapters, none of these thinkers can sustain their arguments for equality as sameness with respect to dietary concerns.

INTERSPECIES EQUALITY AS ASSIMILATION?

The egalitarian arguments for animals mentioned above are *assimilationist* in nature. To count the pain of animals the same as ours, a common animal nature and common interests or needs must be posited. The assumption is that morality requires that we protect or satisfy those common or similar needs *first*; that is, prior to attending to needs that may differ due to the various animals being differently situated by body type, for instance. These arguments for assimilating nonhuman animals disadvantage women and children from two directions: first, by ignoring gender and age differences among humans, and second by ignoring the whole range of body-type and situational differences among the variety of species.

Following what I take to be an assimilationist line, Gary Varner (1994a) has recently argued that virtually all women in the United States are morally required to be vegans because supplements make their risk virtually nil (Varner 1994a). Essentially, Varner is making a "separate-but-equal" or "special-rights" argument. Women and men have separate but "equal" needs. Ethical veganism would not denigrate the moral equality of women (or children) because their requirements are "separate but equally valid." The argument is flawed for two reasons. First, even if risks for vegans are equalized, burdens are not. Western adult male vegans have many fewer burdens to bear while women and child vegans must work harder to be "equal." Adult males rarely suffer anemia; they do not lose iron through periodic menstruation; they do not carry fetuses in their bodies or nurse infants; their growth is completed and they almost always have larger skeletons than females and so have a much lower incidence of osteoporosis. Iron supplements are expensive, are best prescribed by a physician to avoid overdose, are usually not covered by insurance, and may increase a vegan woman's personal and psychological worries. They often cause constipation in those who use them (Ossell 1993); and they are a frequent cause of poisonings in young children (Herbert *et al.* 1990).[5]

Second, the adult male norm remains. Even if it is not too risky for a middle-class infant, child, adolescent, pregnant, lactating, perimenopausal, postmenopausal, or elderly female to be a vegan, that judgment will surely be made from a male-biased perspective of assuming that all those women, children, and seniors can fix, mend, or correct their imperfect bodies as necessary (by supplementation, fortified foods, or eating in special ways) to meet a vegan ideal that is much less burdensome for men. The imperative to supplementation affirms the idea of difference as a lack of being, of incomplete reality that negates the life and value of the feminine (cf. Tuana 1993).

The assimilationist approach to equality in the gender differences debate assumes the norm need not be questioned. In the "speciesism" debate, the interests of animals are to be accommodated by the existing system. Where their interests are the same as ours, humans shall be obligated to protect them. Where they are different, equality has little to say.

Yet, these assimilationist arguments rely on a concept of some common animal nature shared by humans and most other animals capable of experiencing pain or having interests (see chapter 2). In areas that concern differences, the principle of equality conceived on an assimilation model falls apart: which animal should we choose as the paradigm? A fair amount of implicit confusion underlies much of the debate about our duties to animals. For example, probing some arguments uncovers a *human norm* rather than an animal norm. Many animal rights advocates and feminists make an argument from moral respect based loosely on Immanuel Kant's second formulation of the Categorical Imperative: Treat persons always as ends-in-themselves and never as a mere means only. Persons are beings with moral standing, and so animals (by separate argument) are persons. *Ergo*, human beings who use domestic working animals make them solely tools or instruments. In human relations, working for another person is not objectionable because each person consents to the relationship. But because the animals cannot and presumably would not consent to such work, humans are described as using a living being merely as a tool and thus fail to show the animals proper respect. But the argument depends on applying an objectionable human norm to animals. Apparently, even the most humane keeping of cattle could not show moral respect because animals "do not want to be so treated, and we know that" (Donovan 1990, 375). In other words, if domestic animals were rational, they might not consent. But animals do not possess human rationality, so they cannot consent to their relationships with humans. Therefore, *any* use of such animals is wrongful: "without our needing them . . . they would not exist" (Adams 1993, 203). Such arguments assign the very existence of all or virtually all domestic species to *worthlessness*. Yet, moral respect would appear to require humans to treat these animals as having worth, or as the kind of beings *they* are regardless of our expectations. So, reliance on a principle of moral respect falls into inconsistency. Assimilationist thinking aims to circumvent the problem of differences and falls back on understanding interspecies equality in anthropocentric terms. Assuming a species-bridging norm is as futile as assuming a gender-bridging norm for some issues. The assimilation model of equality is inappropriate for deciding about gender differences and is likewise even less useful for adjudicating the treatment of animals. But, the concept of empowerment may be useful in considering species differences and the good of animals.

INTERSPECIES EQUALITY AS EMPOWERMENT?

A second tack would be to use Scales' empowerment model. In interspecies situations we would set aside concerns about assessing species equality and work to diminish domination and emphasize empowerment. Not all uses of animals are properly termed "domination," but domesticated animals have a social nature and their relative docility makes it possible to keep them in wretched conditions. The empowerment model offers promise in curtailing some abusive practices in industrialized agriculture. Restrictive caging of laying hens is objectionable because it frustrates so many of the activities natural to a chicken—the caging disempowers the chicken to do what chickens do. Such chickens can sensibly be regarded as situationally disadvantaged with respect to their free-ranging cousins and related wild birds. So, to be fair to a domestic animal, it should be free enough to display its ordinary species behaviors (see Rollin 1981).

The empowerment model requires that humans study and learn the behaviors of other species. Since animals cannot express their desires in symbolic language, we must communicate with them behaviorally. And, of course, most experienced herders, animal behaviorists, and pet owners do improve their understanding of the needs and desires of their animals over time.

Understanding cannot be equated with empowerment, though. Hunters, too, must understand animal needs and desires in order to be successful. If you agree that trophy hunting or killing an animal purely for sport is wrong (as I do), then in addition to knowing and understanding the behavior of animals, humans also need to integrate *human* values to judge whether interspecies interactions are *fair*. That is, *our* intentions matter. It is not as if we are all animals with the same (or equal) needs and interests. Only humans can argue and try to convince one another to modify "natural" desires and propensities to achieve harmony with other humans and some domesticated species. Some animal species are "wild." Part of the meaning of that term seems to be that humans do not or cannot control the behavior of these animals. Their desires or interests are often opposed to ours. Their *differences* from us may be more extreme. Yet, any eco-ethics must try to recognize these differences and evaluate ways to achieve a fair balance. In fact, difference is perhaps the *sole reason* that ethics is necessary at all. Any ethics must offer ways of governing or encouraging cooperation among competing desires, goals, aims, needs, and interests. We need an ethics that will help us decide when difference is more morally relevant than sameness. In this text, I cannot fully explore such an ethics. At most, I wish to propose some criteria for evaluating interspecies differences. The aim of this book has been to articulate the presuppositions and the "picture" inherent in some traditional and ecofeminist views that makes them incoherent.

The criticisms that I made of the empowerment model hold across species, too. We need to know what kinds of situations and experiences count as domination, disadvantage, or disempowerment for other species. The problem is the empowerment model adds nothing new: *we must already know what constitutes domination and disadvantage before we can equalize empowerment.* But, of course, if disempowerment is wrong and is the same as domination or disadvantage, then the criterion is originally circular and begs the question. Back to square one.

But, it seems to me that the teleological and biological differences across species are greater most of the time between species than within our own. So, one might respond that the empowerment model can work for an interspecies ethics for two reasons: First, we are only able to communicate with other species behaviorally. While it is true that we do assess the interests and the good of animals in ways that include human values, we understand the essential natures of nonhuman animals in more objective terms than we understand what a *human nature* might be. In fact, many thinkers have argued that human beings are constantly creating and revising the nature of what it is to be human. We are actually unable to do otherwise, given our capacities for language and self-critical thought.[6] So, humans have a better understanding of how to treat animals well than they may have concerning other human beings. If this is so, then the empowerment model would not be circular because our knowledge is based on empirical observation and depends less or not at all upon the variety of imaginative self-conceptions individuals or societies may adopt to define their own natures.

Second, if the first claim is true, then the empowerment model may suggest ways to deal with situational differences between or among species. I have argued somewhat briefly that the lives of domestic animals are not expendable and should not be regarded as worthless. To be fair to those who keep domestic breeds alive, would it be acceptable to take their eggs or kill some of the chickens painlessly as long as these birds are kept in acceptable conditions? We can admit that humans do need these birds, but our needing them does not have to be exploitive. The conditions under which they are raised are often deplorable, and we do not need them in the quantity that they are raised now. An empowerment model suggests that our desires be modified to reflect more accurately our *needs* rather than our preferences, and the reason to modify them is to make it possible to raise these chickens in conditions that permit them to *be chickens*.

Interspecies Equality as Acceptance?

Littleton's acceptance model focuses on the function of equality rather than any abstract ideal. Her view avoids reference to any abstract notion of human nature but presupposes that some similarities exist across genders and ages. Thus, in extending the acceptance model to interspecies concerns, we would need a rough notion of similarities in animal behaviors and interests to apply her concept, but no abstract idea of interspecies animal nature is needed. She advises a stepwise approach to evaluating the situations of inequality and to remedying them. Her *methodology* has merit; but, although preferable for issues of gender differences, the acceptance model is probably less appropriate for dealing with interspecies situations. The reasons that the acceptance model is less plausible for applying interspecies equality are based in morally relevant differences among the species.

Some differences are as morally important as similarities if we consider the good of the individual being. Ecofeminist vegetarians often link the oppression of animals with the oppression of women (Adams 1994). But Andrée Collard (1989) remarked that

> 'liberation' . . . is the wrong word to use with reference to animals.
> . . . *True* liberation movements have always started from among the oppressed and have been fuelled by anger, frustration, and yearning to be free . . . from the oppressor's grip *and* from the internalised

perception of the self as victim which keeps the oppressed bound to the oppressor. Liberation is an individual's battle with the pressures of culture, prejudice, and oppression. Animals have no such battle to fight. All they need is freedom from human control (97, italics in original).

Collard points to an important difference between human and nonhuman animals—"the internalised perception of the self as victim." The gap that separates the species looms large because research suggests that self-conception is absent for all nonhumans except perhaps some chimpanzees and related primates (Savage-Rumbaugh and Rumbaugh 1978a,b; Savage-Rumbaugh, Rumbaugh, and Boyson 1978). The gender gap is much narrower, all things considered. Human beings are able to explain to one another the ways in which they feel disadvantaged or dominated. Animals and humans do share certain emotive and behavioral communications about distress and satisfaction, capacities for sociability and play. But, any description or assessment of differences between the species falls unequally on our side and reflects more what we think of ourselves than of them. Such is especially true in a culture whose day-to-day contact with working animals or wild animals is virtually nil and confined to annual visits to the petting zoo or wild animal park. Small wonder in a culture such as ours that most live animals are viewed as pets or threats!

The variety of species is enormous and our relationship with them is equally varied. Some are sacred, others are vermin, still others are useful. Some work with us, some comfort us. Some are simply nuisances and others are dangerous. Some provide food, fur, hide, and fiber for clothing. Some appear beautiful, others grotesque. Some are familiar, others are odd or strange. Yet none of these relationships is static—vermin become pets, totems disappear, human needs change, the strange becomes commonplace. Any relational ethic that attempts to treat other species in proportion to their differences thus faces a daunting task—a task further complicated by the necessity of evaluating their significance in various cultural contexts.

Animals, especially domesticated ones, need something other than "freedom from human control." Domestic species need the humane care and control of humans. They are entitled to that in virtue of our long association and interdependence with them. In my view, the human community is composed of these species as well as our own. All forms of socialization involve some acquiescence to control by others, but such acquiescence does not always constitute oppression or domination if a realization of one's individual good is made possible. "Domination" connotes a form of objectionable control. While it is generally objectionable to place geographic limitations on the travel of adult humans, a fenced playground for a four-year-old child or a fenced range for cattle creates other goods for these beings, such as safety, security, and a degree of freedom appropriate to their experience and intelligence.

The third model, acceptance, functions to question the norm of equality on the deepest level (Littleton 1987). With their voices, with their speech, those humans who hold power define reality, they "speak the world." They define what is to be aspired to, their point of view is accepted as "simple reality." Littleton captures the essence of Collard's point about human versus animal liberation. Humans create and live in an ideational world. Gender and interspecies equality must take root there. Little as humans may like it, we make that "simple reality" within which we and other species co-exist. Only a human being can imagine a world that could be synchronized or harmonized so that everyone has a similar measure of success in satisfying species or individual desires and interests. That sort of world is an ideal world, and while it may never be realized, its value lies in defining what we should strive to achieve if we are to be truly good people.

Some ideals may be self-defeating if they rely on images of human being or the natural world that are incoherent. I have argued here that the "vegan ideal" is an incoherent ideal. As such, it is self-defeating. If we employ it, we may live inauthentically. That is, we may live as if we are what we are not. Under the traditional "vegan ideal," women might try to live as if we did not have the vulnerabilities that we do; we might raise our children that way, too. Individuals might assume that they themselves would not suffer on such diets, only to discover that they have.

Alternatively, using the same "vegan ideal," humans could choose to modify the environment so that people could "move in the direction of vegetarianism." But moving in that direction would have environmental consequences, some of which may also result in unfairness. We need a new ideal, a new picture of ourselves and of the natural world. The ideal world cannot be static. It will respond to the changing structures of the human social world. But it need not be arbitrary. Because other species do not communicate with us in human ways, we will necessarily need to study the typical behaviors of individual species and the particular behaviors of individuals to understand needs and interests. Equality as acceptance, when coupled with the idea of teleological empowerment, could serve as a useful criterion upon which to decide when sameness or difference matters more. Littleton's functionalist approach has value in setting the question: What is equality for, when it concerns other species? The answer should be worked out in a context-to-context approach with the idea of reducing domination. Thus, when such a combined view of equality is implemented, differences among other species and our own should cost less.

In the following chapter, I explore the most current version of feminist ethical vegetarianism—contextual moral vegetarianism. I show why this view is not a morality, and outline my own endorsement of feminist aesthetic semivegetarianism, and a view that incorporates this mixed "empowerment-acceptance" version of equality.

CHAPTER 7

FEMINIST AESTHETIC
SEMIVEGETARIANISM

OVERVIEW

Some feminists have recently suggested a limited version of moral vegetarianism—one that is "contextual" (esp. Curtin 1991, 1992a,b). That is, vegan or vegetarian practice may be required in some contexts but not others. In this final chapter, I revisit contextual moral vegetarianism in order to explain the idea in some detail and to show its intuitive appeal. As a preface to it, I give some general remarks about contextualism. After that, I revisit Deane Curtin's ideas on contextual moral vegetarianism (which I shall refer to as CMV for brevity) and follow it with an explication of the weaknesses of CMV. I show that CMV cannot be classed as a morality because it makes no moral prescriptions and offers no moral guidance. Then, I link together views of equality and difference with the relational contexts of eating alone and eating with others. Finally, I explain why a moderate acceptance of "semivegetarian" diets is most consistent with a balanced moral point of view. Such semivegetarianism has an "aesthetic" basis in nonmoral ideals of personal and global health. Its *limiting factors* are moral because these constraints are feminist caring commitments to equality.

CONTEXTUAL MORAL VEGETARIANISM REVISITED

In chapter 3, I discussed feminist contextual ethics and gave a brief overview of Deane Curtin's views (see his 1991, 1992a,b), which I take to be the best-

149

developed defense of contextual moral vegetarianism. His approach combines virtue ethics, an ethics of care, and an ethics of capability to function (1994, personal communication). Classical virtue ethics was discussed in chapter 2 and an introduction to Curtin's view was given in chapter 3. An ethics of capability to function closely parallels virtue ethics and makes the development of "healthy personhood" the aim of the good life. He argues that the self is discovered in the ordinary experiences of food in daily life. The focus on the ordinary blurs the distinction between the moral and the aesthetic and creates a union of the mind and body through choosing, eating, and experiencing food. The activity of choosing food well affirms the wellness of the self, both spiritually and physically. Rather than envisioning oneself dualistically as an autonomous agent living over against the world, fending off domination by others, the healthy self has "the power to direct one's life [through] accepting herself as body" (1992a, 8). Paying attention to our own personal experiences as we grow, prepare, and eat food enables us to become self-aware and to develop as healthy persons. "We are," he reminds us, "what we eat in a most literal, bodily way. Our bodies literally are food transformed into flesh, tendon, blood, and bone" (11). Healthy people would see themselves in a "participatory" relation with food as self-defining.

One should aim to develop a "healthy personhood." Curtin accepts a plurality of norms and would deny that human beings have an *essential* function or nature. The cultivation of becoming a healthy and good person means finding ways to unify the self and the other, the subject and the object, and to reduce domination over others, whether human or animal. For this reason, eating meat in Western countries is particularly problematic: in "industrialized countries flesh foods are almost exclusively encountered in contexts that express alienation from and dominance over other beings" (Curtin 1992b, 132).[1] The food technology industry objectifies animals. By making them seem distinct from the self, they appear as "other." According to Curtin, becoming a moral vegetarian is an affirmation of an aim *towards* nonviolence.

A *relational* rather than individualistic conception of the self is an important aspect of CMV because it supposedly avoids the rifts of a dualistic perspective (Curtin 1992a). The approach to ethical responsibility and theory-making is what philosopher Lisa Heldke refers to as a *coresponsible option* (1988, 1992a). Heldke explains that the term *coresponsible* "is meant to evoke, among other things, the fact that acting in the world is a communal, relational activity—that we are in correspondence with, and are also responsive and responsible to, others in the world" (1992a, 310). Such an outlook is not completely relativistic because some practices cannot be tolerated, but a variety of perspectives and workable approaches to life problems are validated.

CMV does *not* imply that treating "other animals as food is morally justifiable in exotic cultures, or in the 'Third World,' or in extreme contexts" (Curtin 1992b, 132). But, CMV "is completely compelling as an expression of an ecological ethic of care . . . for economically well-off persons in technologically advanced countries" (Curtin, 1991, 70). Some reasons for this include: "the taking of life should be regarded as a morally serious matter in any culture" (Curtin 1992b, 132), and "the healthful response to food . . . comes from taking only what one needs, and from eating with others in mind" (128). One should affirm "a commitment to eliminate violence wherever possible" (132). "Killing animals for food inflicts needless, conscious suffering" (131) and reducing suffering reduces violence.

CMV cannot be a universal principle (Curtin 1991); it is a "moral direction" to be consciously chosen (Curtin 1992 a,b). CMV parallels the virtue approach in its emphasis on what one *is* rather than what one *does* (Curtin 1994, personal communication). Vegetarianism should not be thought of as a "morally pure high ground" because no one can achieve pure nonviolence (Curtin 1992b, 135). We must kill some living things to eat. CMV is not "universalizable" nor could it be an "absolute moral rule" that could apply "under all circumstances" (Curtin 1992b, 135; 1991, 69). Neither a rule-centered ethics nor an ethics of duty, it most closely resembles an ethics of virtue or well-functioning. CMV is a "direction" to be adopted in keeping with a more general idea that nonviolence is better than violence. Thus, Curtin appears to reject venerating the "vegan ideal."

Many feminists, from the nineteenth century up to the present day, have held that vegetarianism is a political act. Curtin echoes Carol Adams' (1990) claim that "rebuking a meat-eating world is the final state in the vegetarian quest. In its practice vegetarianism rebukes a meat-eating society because it proves that an alternative to meat eating exists and that it works. . . . it rebukes a patriarchal society, since as we have seen meat eating is associated with male power" (1990, 178). Curtin links vegetarianism, political action and character development: Becoming a moral vegetarian can be "seen as a political act of self-empowerment that resists the externalizing pressures of society. To *choose* one's food and define oneself by that choice in opposition to a dominant conceptual scheme is empowering" (1992b, 133, italics in original). Empowerment differs for males and females: For men, "it constitutes a rejection of the disciplinary attempts of meat producers to decide what it means to be a 'real man'. . . . Moral vegetarianism can be understood as a kind of protest" (1992b, 133). And, finally, "it also marks a statement of solidarity with those who resist the oppression of women and nonhuman animals" (1992b, 133).

In summary, Curtin gives several reasons to adopt CMV: (1) it unifies the body and mind to overcome dualisms and dichotomies; (2) choosing food well affirms the spiritual and physical wellness of the self; (3) CMV reduces expressions of dominance and inappropriate uses of power; (4) as a pluralistic ethics of virtue, it avoids essentialism; (5) it affirms a relational view of the self rather than an individualistic one. Finally, Curtin claims (6) practice of it will reduce suffering and violence, furthering a feminist goal of nonviolence. Does CMV succeed in fulfilling these promises? I shall argue that it does not. None of Curtin's goals can be fulfilled by his approach, and in the end the reader will see that Curtin's view is likely to be less effective and less morally consistent than a view that permits some use of meat and animal products but commands humane farming practices.

WEAKNESSES OF CONTEXTUAL MORAL VEGETARIANISM

Curtin makes a number of appealing claims. Unfortunately, some of the claims are mutually incompatible and some claims he simply asserts when he should provide argument. Some of his claims seem plausible because they appeal to our cherished beliefs and traditional connections between vegetarianism, purity, and harmony. Are these connections real or illusion? Some of the connections stretch back two millennia. Some of them are part of a patriarchal system that oppresses women. The following subsections discuss the fallacies and inconsistencies of CMV in its current form.

CMV CONFUSES USE OF POWER WITH WRONGFUL ACTION

Deane Curtin, Carol Adams, Josephine Donovan, Greta Gaard, and many other ecofeminist vegetarians argue that meat eating is wrong because it makes the animal an object. Such objectification is wrong because it is a manifestation of domination. That is, power arises from objectifying the animal as "other." Such objectification is immoral because it is noninclusive, nonegalitarian, fails to consider the suffering of animals, or is exercised out of simple preference for meat rather than any kind of real need. But to avoid circularity in the argument, remember that the question should concern when the uses of power are wrongful. Surely not all exercise of power is dominating. Some are directive, educative, or even defensive. In Curtin's argument here, one infers, nullifying the distinction between self and other is supposed to nullify the power difference and dissolve domination. Let us say that Curtin's strategy is effective and that oneself and the animal become unified, the same—they are equal. Does this immediately entail ethical action, specifically nonviolence? It does not. Another assumption is needed for the inference: that no one would willingly harm herself. However, one *may* do so. And it may even be right to do so. Some uses of power are justified. Ethical standards are used to distinguish the responsible uses of power from the abusive uses. Nondomination cannot, by itself, serve as a foundation for a moral vegan ideal, then, because killing an animal may not be an action of domination, an abuse of power, or a manifestation of oppression. Sometimes killing an animal is the responsible thing to do, as Curtin admits. We need to find deeper criteria for understanding the contexts within which such responsible action may be chosen.

The injunctions against domination of animals by humans forbid cruelty and callousness, even in traditional frameworks. So, should good people adopt vegetarianism as a political act? Curtin answers in the affirmative. As part of healthy personhood one should adopt vegetarianism as "a kind of protest . . . [that] marks a statement of solidarity with those who resist the oppression of women and nonhuman animals" (1992b, 133). He also cites examples of the alienation and objectification that occur in industrialized cultures where people do not associate the meat with the once-living animal. Chickens, swine, cattle, and other domesticated food animals are most often raised in crowded conditions that can only be described as inhumane, and most consumers do not know or care about their plight. One should become a vegetarian to reduce cruelty and abuse, domination and oppression of women and animals.

In response, let us agree that cruelty and abuse of power are wrong because or if these cause pain to the conscious being. Most sorts of "factory farming" conditions should be eliminated primarily because they cause pain or frustration of natural behaviors. But it is very likely possible to raise and slaughter animals in good conditions where such suffering and frustration do not occur. Pain-free slaughter seems to be possible (Grandin 1989a,b). The political action to be taken then becomes advocacy for more humane farming and slaughter, not necessarily vegetarianism.

CMV CONFLATES CONSCIENCE WITH LIBERTY

Moreover, animals cannot be dominated, oppressed, or liberated in the same way that women can be. Domination of women involves an "internalised perception of the self as victim" (Collard 1989, 97). Women have a conception of equality, fairness, and justice. Animals that exist in squalid and crowded conditions may desire to be released, but do not set out to release others from similar conditions. For this reason, the empowerment model of equality as difference is well-suited to understanding how to treat nonhuman animals. Equality should permit animals to function as the kind of beings they are. Nonhuman animals are not (for the most part) ideational beings. Women are. Women have the potential to "speak the world"—to define and create the "simple reality" that is the foundation of meaning and values for the community of humans and animals. So, talking about protesting the similar oppression of women and nonhuman animals confuses the issue. For nonhuman animals, the real issue concerns pain and frustration of their usual natural behaviors. Animals are being treated unethically, but are not being denied *political* voices. For women, the issue is both moral and political—it is wrong or unjust and an abuse of power to disadvantage women, to exclude them from the structure that defines cultural reality, and to make them bear the costs of attempting to live as if they resemble males.

These differences are crucial to the working out of equality and difference. Equality should be viewed functionally, and so we must attend to the fact that animals are differently situated. These differences matter. Tellingly, the specious association of oppression of women and animals weakens CMV. Animals should be empowered to realize their species natures, but humans need freedom to create their individual natures.

EITHER CMV REQUIRES ESSENTIALISM OR CMV HAS NO MORAL CONTENT

Contextual moral vegetarianism as explicated by Curtin suffers from a defect common to most, if not all, modern virtue ethics (see chapter 2). The morality is without content unless some essential human nature, function, or ideal sets the reference point for deciding whether someone has a good or bad character and so has done something right or wrong. Virtue ethics presupposes a common teleological understanding of human excellence; that is, the ethical person must know what she should aim to become. CMV relies on "healthy personhood" as a common aim and a common possibility, and this idea of healthy personhood gives CMV its moral content. Healthy personhood requires essentialism for both theoretical and practical concerns—it serves as a standard for deciding about our own actions and character and about those of others.

As noted in the previous chapter, most feminists object to essentialism— the idea that we share as humans and perhaps as animals, too, some common nature and that this commonality must be most important to deciding how best to treat each other. Empowerment and acceptance views of equality, discussed in the previous chapter, stress the importance of differences. In making differences central to working out equality, such views deny essentialism. So, Curtin would deny that his view is essentialist. But if he does, then he must give up the idea that anyone can aim for healthy personhood. If the contextualist denies that human beings have an essential nature or function, then CMV can project no standard against which to judge whether someone's personhood is healthy or sick (good or evil). Worse yet, if the contextualist persists in claiming a subjective standard (one set for oneself), then the pattern of anyone's flourishing or "healthy personhood" has *no defense beyond her own personal taste.* "Healthy" becomes whatever one might wish it to be, and she must deny that her particular conception of the good extends to anyone else.

Other critics of virtue ethics point out that, without a teleological understanding of human excellence, the person aiming to become moral has no way to unify her moral character and create integrity: actions stand as piecemeal parts of her character without a harmonious pattern (Hittinger 1989). One's character just becomes whatever one has chosen in light of the values she already has or decides to adopt along the way. Without the standard, when people make judgments about actions and character, they are merely reaffirming their already-held beliefs. So, if their beliefs are mistaken, they will never find out using this moral contextualist framework. Moreover, recent work attempting to develop a "free-standing virtue ethic" without specifying a "view of human nature, human society, and the human condition on which [an] argument can be based leaves it floating in air" (Kultgen 1998a, 328; see also Slote 1992).

Curtin's view seems plausible because it appeals to an old framework in updated language. It is appealing because many people tend to accept the idea that peace, harmony, nonviolence, wholeness, and purity are desirable in an ideal world. Many people commonly believe that people should be permitted self-realization and the satisfaction of their preferences. So, a healthy person would want these, too. But that is just what is at issue: Are these commonly held beliefs about what it is to be a *morally* "healthy person" true or at least "fuzzily true"? And does wanting self-realization, peace, harmony, nonviolence, wholeness, and purity necessarily require vegetarianism, or does it just seem so because these ideas have been joined to vegetarianism in an appealing way?

CMV Requires a Discriminatory Vegan Ideal

CMV would endorse moving in a direction towards moral vegetarianism wherever possible on grounds that a healthy person would desire the reduction of violence towards animals, resolution of dualities, and equalization of power. Practically speaking, this amounts to holding up a vegan ideal, even though Curtin says it should not. To see this, let's think about an example. Suppose we live in a world where everything in the natural world is the same as it is now, but human social institutions have been rearranged to be fairer. Part of this conception of fairness is that those who can do so will adopt a contextual moral vegetarianism. The society is composed of real people like you and me. Some people won't be as responsible as others. Some will compete to be better (more "saintlike") than others. Some may even be rebellious and compete for the "demonic." The middle group will take their responsibilities most seriously and try to put their beliefs into action most consistently. They will also try to convince the irresponsible ones to change their ways. Now, I think that in this society, if women and children have the *will* to succeed, they can have as much success in taking these actions as men. The evidence for this lies in populations around the world today, where more women than men are, in fact, vegetarians. In this imaginary society, let us suppose, equal numbers of men and women would achieve "healthy personhood." But fewer of the women (as well as children and others named earlier) would achieve optimum physical health, and some would suffer ill *physical health* because of it—effects that their adult male vegetarian counterparts would not have to suffer. If, on the other hand, some or many women reject vegetarianism as a moral direction on nutritional grounds, males are sure to be seen as more virtuous and more physically perfect than females, children, and others. If women accept the practice, the physical disadvantages between the genders and age groups will be exacerbated, offering further fuel to the notion of feminine inferiority.

CMV RELIES ON JUDGMENTS OF TASTE

Before I begin my critique in this section I want to make a distinction between moral appeals and aesthetic ones. Curtin calls his view a "contextual *moral* vegetarianism." In a traditional ethical system, aesthetic appeals are opposed to moral commands. Curtin is using the word "moral," but he clearly wants to avoid appealing to traditional moral systems. Curtin is appealing to a more blended version of aesthetic/moral. Even so, the words have to be tied to their original meaning in some sense. In a traditional system, some aesthetic claims are just arbitrary. You like custard pie, and I like boysenberry pie. It's just a matter of personal preference. Boysenberry pie reminds me of my childhood because we had rows and rows of thorny berry vines that we picked, all the while eating as much as we picked. And Mom would make pies and jam. This is all very nice but has nothing to do with morality, of course. It's just my taste. I wouldn't *be required* to like the berry pie. Other aesthetic judgments appeal to a more or less objective standard, perhaps an intersubjective standard, of beauty or goodness. The works of Michelangelo are aesthetically beautiful independent of whether you or I like them or not. The traditional moral theorist divides the moral and the aesthetic in this way, and the aesthetic is further divided into judgments of goodness and judgments of taste. A judgment of taste is one that has no justification beyond one's own personal preference, and basing one's moral decisions judgments of taste is objectionable.

Now, recall or look back to the section above entitled "Either CMV Requires Essentialism or CMV Has No Moral Content." There I showed that CMV must rely on essentialism for its coherence—the idea that there is some definite human nature. But the pattern of anyone's flourishing or "healthy person-hood" has no defense beyond her own personal likes and dislikes, the values she already has. So, the view becomes arbitrary and morally objectionable if any-thing could count as "healthy personhood." Curtin clearly does not think just anything at all could count. But is he right? Proponents of CMV tend to try to convince others to accept their view, so they apparently do not *intend* to be arbitrary. But, simply intending not to be arbitrary does not make it so. CMV would not be arbitrary if the aim is aesthetic but intersubjectively defensible. If one asks: *You* may like this version of "healthy personhood," but why should I? The reason you should like it, too, lies in self-fulfillment rather than morality. Focusing on the ordinary everyday experiences of food and its preparation, Curtin claims, blurs the distinction between the moral and the aesthetic and unifies the mind and body. The vegetarian becomes "embodied spirit." A healthy self has the power to direct her own life by "accepting herself as body" (Curtin 1992a, 8). Curtin appeals to common desires for unity, harmony, and self-realization. An appeal to a common human nature is also assumed, but perhaps Curtin would assent to that after all. The question becomes, Has he succeeded in making a moral rather than an aesthetic claim?

While feminists often argue for the resolution of dichotomies such as mind/body, Curtin does not show that moral/aesthetic is a distinction that *should* become blurred. In fact, blurring it creates other problems. At the very least, morality should give guidance concerning our relationships with others, guid-ance about when to thwart our own desires as well as when to gratify them. Blurring the distinction between the moral and the aesthetic blurs our ability to decide which desires may be "healthy" for us but cause "illness" in others.[2] Blurring this distinction makes CMV a subjective working out of one's already held preferences and then acting to satisfy them. In traditionalist language, this is just simple egoism, an old and very appealing idea dressed up in new words.[3] But it is not virtue or goodness; it is simply cloaked selfishness.[4]

Moreover, these aesthetic judgments are matters of personal preference. One who adopts vegetarianism because she prefers the taste of vegetables, the look of them, the way she feels when she eats them, or perhaps from a sense of communion with nature or to make herself alive with their life also gives aesthetic rather than moral reasons for her choices. It makes her *feel* good, but does it make her *be* good? And if it makes her be good, that good must be relational, not simply with the way she feels about and treats *herself* but with the way she feels about and treats you and me. Neither Curtin nor Carol Adams would claim aesthetic reasons as the most important reasons to adopt vegetarianism, but take away these "positive benefits" and consider the discrimination and bias that I have exposed in the vegan ideal and CMV looks much less convincing.

In the end, I think that Curtin is arguing for adoption of a nonmoral "aesthetic preference-interest" (see chapter 3). These interests are associated with goods that will benefit the person herself. They are not virtues that *any* person ought to adopt to have a good moral character. Virtues or moral character traits, such as courage and truthfulness, are characteristics of all good persons. Nonmoral traits make you a pleasing (or pleased) person, but not a *morally good* one. Curtin has confused a nonmoral psychological trait with a moral one. Thus, he loses the basis for calling his view a moral one.

CMV GAINS APPEAL BY ASSOCIATION WITH PURITY

Much of the appeal of CMV relies on positive associations held over from a more patriarchal worldview. As noted in chapter 2, vegetarianism in the nineteenth century and in the 1970s was a spiritual movement founded on an "ethic of naturalness." Many of Curtin's claims for CMV echo vegetarian purist ideals, and Carol Adams' endorsement of vegetarianism also appears to be heavily reliant on a traditional nonmoral aesthetic preference for purity, a "virtue" always ascribed to ideal women. Vegetarians were and still are predominantly women. Women have been symbolized as closer to nature and givers of life. In the "ethic of naturalness," meat—"steak dripping with blood"—is rejected as symbolic of death, blood being the ultimate taboo (Twigg 1979; cf. Adams 1990, 185). Only vegetarian food is "pure."

Although vegetarians adopt their diet in an attempt to resolve mind/body dualities, the dualities of human nature become exacerbated in the structure of vegetarian symbolic behaviors. That is, vegetarians wish to become, as Curtin would put it, "embodied spirit," but in the process become unable to accept the reality of the body that experiences violence, good and evil, suffering, and eventual death. How does this happen? Let's reconstruct the chain of dualistic associations that have survived since Pythagoras. First, flesh is representative of one's "lower bodily nature" as opposed to the "higher" rational, spiritual, and moral soul. Only the body dies; the spirit cannot die. The body is the source of desires such as hunger, thirst, sex drive, and other drives that may be violent and destructive. The most *real* nature of human beings is the spirit because spirit permits us to attain the higher virtues by controlling, reducing, and even eliminating the bodily passions. The body and its destructive hungers are unreal (Pythagoras) or less real (Plato, Descartes) than the spirit. The spirit is the essence of the human, and the spirit is good—pure and immortal—rather than evil. Thus, cruelty and aggression are not "natural" to human beings. How did we become cruel and aggressive then? The vegetarian subtly argues that these are brought on by culture, "by a distorting society and a distorted way of eating—the carnivorous" (Twigg 1979, 21).[5] Nineteenth century vegetarians believed that eating animals makes people violent like animals (Twigg 1979, 20). In a similar vein, Adams (1990) struggles to connect slaughter and meat eating by men with the rape and physical abuse of women. Meat is rejected because, in eating an animal one takes in the animal's nature. We encounter our own animal nature and the "constructed barrier between men and beasts" becomes broken (Twigg 1979, 20). Meat is only body, and it is body that can die. Thus, meat is associated with death rather than life. Vegetarian food is "alive as the universe is alive . . . filled with the same life as the trees, the plants, the waving grain" (Twigg 1979, 25). Eating meat is "eating corpses . . . the ingestion of dead animals is an ingestion of death itself" (25). And in Adams (1990), "in experiencing the nothingness of meat, one realizes that one is not eating food but dead bodies" (175; see also 177 for the association of meat with corpses).[6]

Thus, human nature is the spiritual aspect, and only the *"pre-social"* self is natural and good. Moreover, nature is seen as essentially harmonious, bountiful, and beneficent. If this is true, then it follows that people who want to be good and moral will attempt to harmonize the self with nature. Symbolically, vegetarianism rejects death and offers a "this-worldly" salvation of the body. A New Moral Order idealizes the re-establishment of a sort of "Garden of Eden" where the dichotomies of life are resolved into a state of natural harmony.

By now, you will have no doubt noticed that this symbolic structure is thoroughly Cartesian, even though feminist vegetarians would not wish to accept a Cartesian framework! It seems to embrace rather than resolve mind/body, nature/culture dualities. Vegetarians who argue from this framework idealize nature and human nature—see them as they *cannot* be—and then use that ideal to criticize other people and society. Although recent feminist vegetarians criticize patriarchy and call for a "New Moral Order," that new order is based on an old dualistic ideal: "Vegetarian activities counter patriarchal consumption and challenge the consumption of death. Feminist vegetarian activity declares that an alternative worldview exists, one which addresses life rather than consuming death; one which does not rely on resurrected animals [consumed by us] but empowered people" (Adams 1990, 185). Yet, in accepting the symbolic structure above, feminist vegetarians unwittingly embrace patriarchal dichotomies such as the apposition of nature/culture and body/spirit. The rending of nature/culture is problematic because, if culture is seen as unreal, false, unnatural, oppressive, divisive, and distorting, whereas nature is seen as real, pure, raw, natural, free, good, unified, and harmonious, then the vegetarian can no longer understand the suffering, violence, social strife, human vanity, war, cruelty, and death that are a part of our everyday experience. The vegetarian ideology extracts the evil of death and violence away, *defining* it as unreality and placing it outside of the system. The remainder—the spiritual, pre-social self— is good, harmonious, alive, and ultimately "real."

Deane Curtin's CMV avoids many of the pitfalls above because he emphasizes food practice. Yet, his association of nonviolence with vegetarianism suggests reliance on the dichotomy he wishes to resolve. The true embodied spirit must come to grips with the reality of our bodies, of suffering and death in order to live as coresponsible beings. CMV and other forms of feminist vegetarianism build on historic efforts to strike down an aristocratic social order, replacing it with an egalitarian social harmony where the lion lies down with the lamb. But the lion will eat the lamb, for it must. And so sometimes must we.

CMV RELIES ON ANOTHER FALLACY: CHOICE AND CHANCE

Curtin's view of CMV commits a fallacy of confusing bodily health with moral health. I think Curtin courts confusion when he speaks of "healthy personhood." The obvious analogy is bodily health. He does want unification of the body and mind, so that both would function well. And perhaps a fair amount of the appeal of associating vegetarianism with healthy personhood comes from the health benefits for many vegetarians. But, moral health requires decision making and choice in a way not required for bodily health. First, bodily health does not always require that one choose any particular action. Some people are just healthy, even in the face of habits that should be detrimental. Moral health never occurs by accident. One cannot achieve a good character without being taught. One must know the right values and the right ways of acting. Furthermore, one must *choose* to live in accord with those values. Sometimes people know what is right, but choose to do wrong anyway. People are always free to do evil, but good people restrain themselves or develop desires to do good rather than evil. Talking about a "healthy character" is confusing because

we could forget that people get this kind of character by thoughtful deliberation and choice about doing the right thing. And with careful thought, a good
teacher, a good will, and practice over time, most, if not all, human beings can
achieve this kind of a good moral character even with sick bodies.

Having good physical health is another matter. The body will not always
obey. Even the unwavering practice of exercise, good diet, regular checkups,
and every other preventive measure cannot guarantee good health. One may
get sick anyway.[7] But people do not lose their moral health except by acts of
will. A good moral character can only be eroded by choice and not by chance.

Thus, no necessary connection exists between the health of one's moral
character and the health of one's body. Because vegetarianism is particularly
healthy for adult males in industrialized countries, it is tempting to think that
vegetarianism leads to health of the soul—a recurrent idea in most vegetarian
communities all the way back to the Pythagoreans. Many people long for such
unity and harmony, but it might be just as true that conflict and opposition
produce growth and flourishing, virtue and high character.

Basically, Curtin proposes that contextual moral vegetarianism will be
good for the person herself. The underlying motivation is an aim towards nonviolence as the defining characteristic of her wholeness and goodness. But it is
not enough to base a morality upon the good of the self. A benefit to the self is
a nonmoral good, but a moral good is tied to some understanding of a human
good that extends beyond the self alone. Why so? The world is full of good and
evil things that one might desire or, worse, be forced to choose among. Sometimes we cannot choose anything that is good at all! The person of high character knows what action to choose that will further not only her own good but
that of those others whom she affects in choosing. If she must choose to do
something that is simultaneously good and evil, she will know why. And what
if it were true that only by choosing against her own "healthy personhood"
could she further the well-being of her child? How could the criterion of healthy
personhood then serve as the foundation for a morality?

A Tangled Web

Curtin does appear to see some problems with his view. Vegetarianism may aid
in developing a healthy personhood, but it may not, he admits. It all depends
on context. I find this unsatisfying. As I have argued above, his view seems
essentialist and excessively subjective. Worse yet, his view also denies human
freedom. Context itself appears to form the character and not the human will.
If contextual moral vegetarianism does contribute directly to virtue or healthy

personhood, then another, more submerged value is actually at work forming goodness of character. And it may have nothing to do with diet at all. Certainly, the aim toward nonviolence may point to that underlying value. But first one should ask: Should we pursue nonviolence almost always or as one of the foundational virtues? Frankly, although I would say that many modern industrialized contexts are appropriate places for valorizing nonviolence, I also realize that the context for that can change from moment to moment. There are times when women must be ready to fight. Being victims will not improve our characters. Do the contexts drive that change in attitude? Or is it a deeper commitment that carries us across contexts to change our actions? I argue that it is the latter: The will to live by the more fundamental value of equality is the fulcrum to a choice between nonviolence or aggressive defense. Feminists may desire that no one ever suffer pain, violence, or death at the hands of others, yet at the same time feminists must affirm their own lives, the lives of other women, of our children, their health, and their freedom. Only that affirmation will lift us out of victimization. If we choose nonviolence at the expense of well-being, then we choose to be victimized. We must drive the contexts by our values and our choices. The contexts should not drive us.

FEMINIST AESTHETIC SEMIVEGETARIANISM

We must rethink the structure of our views on ethics and equality. What is ethics for? What is equality for? Their function is more relevant than their ontology. I cared about ethical vegetarianism because I am a teacher and a mother. I taught the arguments to my students, who could also think them through for themselves. I accepted ethical vegetarianism myself. I wondered what to teach my daughter, as well as what to feed her. At ten years of age, she was much less capable of thinking through such arguments. If I were to move from context to context on a personal quest to develop my own healthy personhood, making choices in the moral direction of vegetarianism and nonviolence, perhaps ethics would mean something different for me than it does now. But I take a pragmatic view: What is ethics for in the context of my relationship to my family, my students, and the animals who are part of my life? How can I make equality real for them? If I succeed in giving my child the means to become a virtuous, healthy, thoughtful person, what should I have taught her when she was ten years old? What should I teach her now when she is twenty-three? In my view "moral" or "ethical" must be conceptually linked to guidance with respect to our relations with others. Although we guide by example, human beings must also learn by instruction. When we instruct, we make choices and express concerns about behaviors, actions, rules, virtues and ideals. I want to teach my daughter to be good and healthy. Shall I teach her that adopting a moral direction towards vegetarianism is a part of virtue?

Below I explicate the answer I have come to accept, what I refer to as a feminist aesthetic semivegetarianism. I explore some of the contexts within which we eat and suggest ways of evaluating these particular contexts. Like Curtin, I affirm the value of health, but I reject the idea that it can properly be a moral value. Instead, health is an intersubjective aesthetic norm that is better understood with respect to bodily well-functioning than mental or spiritual wellness. We know how to cure anemic blood, but we are less certain about how to cure anemic souls. We should recognize that our prescriptions about vegetarianism are aesthetic and may not apply to others in other contexts. Instead of condemning meat eating, I think it would be more productive (that is, pragmatic) to improve conditions for animals and to urge truly balanced diets that are not excessive. Depending on context, eating small amounts of meat is appropriate, but limited by the moral considerations prohibiting cruelty, violence, and waste. Raising and killing animals in conditions of frustration of natural behaviors or of pain and suffering is morally wrong in any case.

I also incorporate three assumptions: First, there is no universal human norm against which to measure human virtue. Second, women, children and many other groups have different nutritional needs from adult males that make it more burdensome for them to be vegetarians. Third, in a patriarchal world any recommendation about diet must consider the subordinate place and value of women (and children and others) in society as well as the gendered nature of caring work such as food preparation. Politicizing ethics means that recommendations about moral norms must take account of the imbalance of power and make efforts to make differences cost less.

Some of the contexts within which we eat include eating alone, eating with other adults, eating in families, and eating with children. I will discuss these relational contexts, but contexts for eating may be defined by other perimeters such as religious or celebratory events that involve communities. I shall not discuss these here and will leave them for future discussion.

CONTEXTS FOR EATING

The contexts proposed below are exploratory and based on the idea that people live together and influence one another. The idea of "family" should be construed broadly. Almost any group of people can constitute a family. The contexts described below are meant to serve as examples rather than as case parameters.

It is not the context that determines how we should act but the needs and will of the people and nonhuman animals within those contexts.

EATING ALONE

Considering oneself alone and eating without others present, any adult might choose a diet in industrialized countries from veganism to semivegetarianism. Prudence dictates that individuals consider their personal health when deciding on diet. Reasons to take care of ourselves are not simply egocentric. If we do not do so, then we may become overly dependent on others, either for personal care or through use of the health care system. CMV works well, it seems to me, for westernized adults seeking to salvage a spiritual connection between themselves and the world in personal terms. That spiritual connection may improve oneself and be good, but it will be a personal and aesthetic good assessed in a highly individualized context that is not meant to guide others and is neither moral nor immoral. If we eat alone and in privacy, you or I might choose to be vegetarians from the belief that nonviolence in our own lived context is good. But, it would wrong others to count vegetarian diets as *morally* better. On the other hand, because the lives and suffering of animals count, an individual in a society with agriculture would find it more difficult to claim that a heavy meat-eating diet is permissible. But, a person might say to himself or herself: "It will be better if I become a vegetarian. My body will function very well on this diet at my stage of life and in the circumstances that I live. I know, too, that it will spare the lives of the animals I might otherwise eat, and their suffering matters. I choose this diet only if none of my responsibilities for other humans or animals will be compromised by my choosing it. I will not exalt this choice to an ideal nor call it a rule to be generally followed. If I am among people who treat their animals well, I will not claim that my choice should be an example for any other, nor will I press others to follow me in my choice, nor shame them should they continue to eat meat or animal products. And I choose this that I may become a better person." The "better person" in this case fits a personal image of the self that can involve an ideal of personal virtue or function. But one might realize his or her own individual good or perfection and know that she is not realizing a *moral* ideal. It is properly called an aesthetic ideal.

On the other hand, another person might experience the world differently. She or he might not feel as confident about her health (for instance, she might have allergies or be pregnant or live where there are few fresh vegetables and so forth). She might choose to eat enough meat, milk, and eggs to be sure that she is maintaining her health, balancing her good with the good of the lives of her human and nonhuman companions. She therefore chooses semivegetarianism. In fairness, with respect to what she eats, she and her vegetarian counterpart are equally good. The moral aspect of one's character has to do with one's relations with others. In this case, the good person permits others to choose the right diet for themselves, limited only by semivegetarian constraints. However, nothing forbids the individual from educating others without vegetarian proselytizing about the conditions food animals are raised in, the improvements possible with free-range farming, the general safety of semivegetarianism as well as the precautions necessary, and so forth. These efforts can be defended on humanitarian and health grounds.

Feminist aesthetic semivegetarianism *permits* everyone to eat a certain small amount of meat, dairy products and other animal products as long as animals are well treated and killed as painlessly as possible. It respects a somewhat fuzzy boundary of the moral in this way. That is the prohibition against cruelty and violence *limits* how much one may consume. Yet *that* one consumes the meat and animal products is itself aesthetic because it is permitted as a matter of taste, health, and context. Each person must decide the divide between the aesthetic and the moral on the basis of her own conscience alone but setting the line too low (veganism) will often be just as wrongful as setting it too high (excessive meat-eating). So, my differences with Curtin are mostly pragmatic. If you call a practice "moral," as in CMV, then you are committed in some sense to praise and blame, to admonishing and urging conformity. I argue that it is unfair to urge vegetarianism, although I do think people should "eat with others in mind," as Curtin says. Therefore, people ought to follow semivegetarianism. Within that, the degree of abstinence from meat is chosen on the basis of context and preference—anything from veganism to including small amounts of meat regularly.

EATING WITH OTHERS

What should this individual do if she finds herself among others? It seems most consistent to me that she should practice a semivegetarian diet or at least defer to it. Some people really do not wish to consume meat, but there are various symbolic ways to affirm the efforts of pregnant women and parents to provide adequate nutrition to their children through food rather than supplements, for instance. The strict vegetarian might still cut meat for a child.

The good person should not place herself in a position of assuming that she knows or understands the motives and needs of others. For instance, we often do not know the food allergies of our friends much less of the person sitting next to us in a restaurant.[8]

EATING IN FAMILIES

Women and their families live in various contexts. Many families are amalgams of the young and the old, male and female, two or more cultures, two or more species. Families may have many reasons for serving different kinds of food that involve the nutritional needs of its members, health concerns, cultural traditions, and so on. For this example, let us say that our family consists of an adult, a child, and an elderly person. Eating a small amount of meat and using dairy products is defensible for all. Several reasons support this. The first is health; semivegetarian diets are healthy and involve few, if any, of the risks in vegetarian diets. Second, children tend to imitate their parents. If a mother and grandmother do not eat meat or drink milk, then her daughter may not, even if at the daughter's stage of life she is building bones whereas the mother is not. The grandmother may lose bone from inadequate calcium in her diet and become dependent upon the family for care. If a father is not eating any meat or milk, then his son may not even though he too needs to build bone and maintain iron levels.

One might think that each person in the family above should eat according to his or her stage of life. I could not support this for two reasons in addition to those above. In a patriarchal society, women still do most of the food preparation and provisioning (DeVault 1991). Even in households where males share in or do most of the cooking, women are expected to provide all sorts of other caring labors that place them at the center of feeding the family. It would be even more unfair to require women to assume the burden of providing nutritionally balanced meals for several different people at a variety of stages of life.

Second, vegetarianism is especially suitable for adult males. But, in a society where males have most of the power, valorizing vegetarianism for males will only continue to underwrite that power. It could easily be seen as a sign of superior health, physical power and perfection to live as a vegetarian. Every major religion has vegetarian sects within it and has idealized the vegetarian life, possibly since the dawn of agriculture. Thus, it is not unrealistic to suppose that present day values could be inverted to the continued detriment of women, children, and others.

EATING AND PARENTING

Providing meals for children presupposes a special responsibility. Suppose you are trying to decide whether to put your newly weaned, one-year-old daughter on a vegan diet. If you monitor the diet carefully and use supplementation, this is a relatively low risk choice in the United States. Still, there is some risk, and the risk is higher than for adults. Unlike adults, infants and children cannot choose for themselves. If you make the wrong choice, your child will suffer. Let us say that you have read the reviews cited here. You know the importance of iron to your infant's neurological development and calcium to her skeletal development. You could rely on vitamin drops. You are probably giving them to her anyway since most infants get them. Will avoiding certain food sources mean the loss of a significant source of nutrients? It undoubtedly will. Can you replace those nutrients in the food choices you have left? With "careful planning" you can (Jacobs and Dwyer 1988; Dwyer 1991; Dwyer and Loew 1994; Havala and Dwyer 1988, 1993). You also know that the American Academy of Pediatrics (1992) recommends that milk remain a part of children's diets. Your vegetarian cookbook prefers not to recommend vegan diets for infants and children (Robertson *et al.* 1986, 417–18). Must you give her a vegan diet? No. You may be *permitted* to give her a vegan diet if you exercise all precautions, but you cannot be morally required to do so.

Why so? Choosing benefits or safety for others differs from choosing them for ourselves even if the general risks were the same for women and men, the old and the young. Some feminist vegetarians have argued that if the risks are the same then parents must make their children vegans, too (Adams 1995; Varner 1994a,c). But, these arguments conflate what it is *safe* to do with what one must do to be *morally good.* Simply that an action involves low or no risk is not the sole deciding factor. An adult may rationally refuse to take low risk actions. Bungee-jumping involves much lower risk than driving a car, yet it is not irrational to refuse to bungee-jump. For morality, this is not a fair example, of course. Your bungee-jump doesn't risk the health of other people. Making the *right* choice (whether the choice is based on principle, caring, virtue, or function) for others requires that the decisionmaker provide a measure of protection. One should not impose any greater risk than the person herself would wish to take if she were able to decide. Getting into the perspective of the dependent person is required.

To see how having even a small risk imposed on someone else can be objectionable, consider nuclear power generation. Formerly, policymakers and utility companies would assure the public that these plants are safe and that risks are extremely small. They would wave away the concerns of environmentalists and try to build the plants near population centers. But people rightly may have a different concern about very small risks *imposed* upon them versus very serious risks that they choose for themselves. So, part of the objection to nuclear plants can be that the risk imposed on the plant's neighbors is chosen for them by others.

Ethical vegan parents in industrialized countries might reason another way; that is, if their infants or children *were* moral agents, they too would be required to take the risk. Therefore, parents are required to choose the risk for the child.[9] However, parents cannot reasonably be required to adopt any strategy that is deemed low risk for their children unless the benefits significantly outweigh the risk. For example, suppose that a toddler has a chronic disease that might be cured by undergoing a somewhat risky surgery. But the surgeons admit that even under the best conditions serious side-effects can occur. Alternatively, parents can choose a long-term program of treatment that has known outcomes but does not cure. Let us say it is a diet-modification and medication plan that is effective nearly all of the time and causes virtually no ill effects. A cure is *ideally* preferable because once accomplished, the quality of the child's life is improved.[10] If offered such a choice for oneself, *adults* might rationally choose either therapy (or reject both on grounds of self-determination). On the other hand, when choosing for a child, notice that the more conservative diet and medication plan assures that no disastrous results will occur. So, it is permissible that parents opt for the conservative approach; they would not be obligated to take the riskier path. Similarly, with general food practice, it makes a very big difference in choosing *for others* if doing nothing (or maintaining, say, a semivegetarian diet) is likely to produce *no harm at all* whereas adopting a vegan diet carries some risks. There is no evidence that semivegetarian diets are risky for infants or children (Havala and Dwyer 1988), and semivegetarian diets are likely to be less dependent on supplementation than vegan diets. The traditionalist ethical vegetarian position requires that parents take these risks for their children and put them on vegan diets.[11] But this is to confuse what it is safe to do with what one is morally required to do. Feminist aesthetic vegetarianism would leave it to individual parents to decide whether it is appropriate to move in the direction of moral vegetarianism for a child.

SUMMARY

Does my view mean that people can go on eating meat without concern? No, it does not. Absolutism functions only as an attempt at domination; that is, accept this rule and you won't be required to think ever again! Many good reasons exist to moderate our eating habits to semivegetarian practice. These reasons should count with all of us, and we must decide for ourselves what sort of balance is possible in our own lives.

All things considered—the needs of women and children, the tendencies of young females towards eating disorders, pressures on women to diet in general, the extra burden that is placed on women in preparing different kinds of food for each family member, the conditions under which animals are raised—families and people in general should be semivegetarians. We should write, teach, and actively work for a reduction in animal cruelty, to improve the conditions under which animals are raised, to encourage gratitude for their association with us, and to recognize their membership in a community with us. We should not eat them wastefully but only in a portion that balances the needs of family members sharing the same meal. Feminists need not necessarily drop their vegan or vegetarian lifestyles if they and their families are doing well and living happily on them. But I do think feminists must stop preaching the vegetarian life as a moral imperative. Vegetarianism is not morally required. It is an aesthetic choice that may be personally satisfying and healthful. To argue otherwise is divisive and self-defeating.

Because needs vary, feminist aesthetic semivegetarianism does not prescribe measured amounts of meat or dairy products. But, people in most industrialized countries should drastically reduce their consumption of meat and dairy products. Three of the best reasons to endorse a drastic reduction, but not elimination, in meat eating and dairy use are (1) preserving personal health, (2) establishing a global sustainable environment that produces a long-term supply of adequate food, and (3) restoring domestic animals to a place of greater respect by giving them housing, care, transport, and slaughter that empowers these domestic species to their natural activities. Their lives and suffering count and should not be wasted. Efforts at producing global health require attention to the particular contexts of climate, culture, soils, species, and their systems. A balancing of various goods and interests will be necessary, and preaching the evils of meat eating is more likely to do harm than good.

Traditionalist arguments for ethical vegetarianism collapse because they violate their own central Principle of Equality. If we believe that sexism is wrong and women and men should be equal, then we must *accept* speciesism—animals cannot be the equals of humans because women, men, children, and others have differing nutritional needs. But if we *reject* speciesism, then we must *accept* sexism and the belief that women cannot be the equal of men because their bodies are weaker, vulnerable, and inferior to that of adult males, who can practice vegetarianism with relatively little risk. In the face of this dilemma, traditional moral arguments for the rights and welfare of animals are inconsistent and fail. So, these traditional moral arguments for ethical vegetarianism cannot be integrated into a feminist ethic.

Moreover, specifically feminist arguments for ethical vegetarianism or the vegan ideal also fail. The historical and claimed theoretical link between vegetarianism and feminism is a chimera. The vegan ideal is not at all a feminist ideal. Even the feminist arguments assume that the human norm is male, and women are expected to accommodate themselves to it. I have argued that feminist ethical frameworks have been committed to two basic beliefs that I call the "minimum conception of a feminist ethics." These two beliefs are: First, no ethics can admit of arbitrariness in its prescriptions and theories. Second, any specifically feminist ethic must affirm the value of the female body. Current feminist arguments for ethical vegetarianism would require women to live as if physiologically identical to men and assign arbitrary moral or physical burdens to women, children, and others based on factors that cannot be changed by human choice. Thus, the minimum conception rules out ethical vegetarianism. Therefore, my arguments show that all formulations of ethical vegetarianism, whether traditionalist or feminist, fail.

The "vegan ideal" is not a *moral* ideal at all. It may be adopted as a personal lifestyle, but it cannot be a moral ideal because it would idealize those of a particular age, sex, class, ethnicity, and culture; that is, adult (age 20–50), middle-class, mostly white males living in high-tech societies—the group with the most power in our world.

Feminists should not moralize about food practice, even though it remains appropriate to condemn cruelty and to encourage moderation and semivegetarianism for that reason. Equality remains a central principle of any feminist ethic. Reinterpreting equality to include differences suggests that we should adopt equality on a range from empowerment to acceptance. We should work to understand domesticated animal behaviors and to empower their natures within the human-animal relationship and simultaneously attempt to understand and contribute to acceptance as equality among humans. Certainly, sustained discussion and debate will be necessary in order to determine ways to make these differences cost less for those who live them. Because even Deane Curtin's feminist contextual moral vegetarianism collapses to values clarification and offers no moral guidance, individuals must not focus on vegetarianism as an avenue to moral virtue. Instead, we must look again at how to make ethics and equality *functional.* An aesthetic semivegetarianism *permits* everyone to eat a certain small amount of meat, dairy products and other animal products as long as animals are well treated and killed as painlessly as possibly. It respects a fuzzy boundary between the aesthetic and the moral in this way. That is, the imperative *against* cruelty and violence *limits* how much one may consume. Yet *that* one consumes the meat and animal products is itself aesthetic because it is *permitted* as a matter of taste, health, and context. Each person must decide the divide between the aesthetic and the moral on the basis of her own conscience, but depending on those with whom one eats setting the line too low (veganism) will often be just as wrongful as setting it too high (excessive meat eating). We must fashion our diets within social settings, realizing that personal and global health are intersubjectively valid aesthetic values. In some cases it may be that a person will choose vegetarianism or veganism because that choice will most beautify her life. In more ordinary cases, though, feminists should choose aesthetic semivegetarianism in recognition of the differences among males and females, young and old, humans and nonhumans, and those in other cultures and classes, in an effort to *live* equality as acceptance, and in affirmation of personal and global health as well as strength of character as guiding values.

NOTES

CHAPTER 1—INTRODUCTION

1. My narrative here of the rise of individual liberty omits certain important assertions that many feminists associate with it. Ecofeminists, in particular, associate individual liberty with man-centered thinking, instrumentalism, loss of community, exploitation of nature, animals, women, and vulnerable classes as well as the devaluation of the feminine. These objections have merit. On the other hand, so-called "liberal ideals" forced society to recognize the equality of women and to affirm the intrinsic value of life and nature.

2. Vice is the technical contrast to virtue, thus, the adjective "vicious." Today, we usually do not apply such terms to persons of bad character, preferring instead to medicalize their aberrations as "sick." This may be indicative of a gradual change in the character of our ordinary everyday moral judgments.

3. See Singer (1975, 181), where he argues for the vegan lifestyle as most virtuous, although he encourages a less stringent vegetarianism as a practical beginning towards this ideal.

4. For example, Lori Gruen (1993) reports that the Ecofeminist Task Force requested that the National Women's Studies Association adopt a policy of serving only vegan meals at its 1991 conference and all future conferences as a strong statement of feminist nonviolence (see also Adams 1994).

5. The most important exception to this is, of course, David Hume, who argued for sentiment or "fellow feeling" as the ground for ethical thought.

6. An objectionable hierarchy is associated with designating some cultures as "first" and others as "third" or at any other numerical degree. However, other terms such as "developed" or "underdeveloped" seem even more objectionable; I have also found it necessary to use the term "developing" later to paraphrase cited authors.

7. The term "blind" here is a technical term; it should be viewed in the positive sense of enabling the scientist to discover something apart from her own personal interests, goals, and prejudices. I apologize to anyone who finds any metaphorical use of the term offensive, but alternative terms are not available.

8. These conclusions are drawn primarily from studies of American Seventh-Day Adventists.

9. Most positions require other actions (such as abstinence from smoking and alcohol, for example) in addition to vegetarianism, but I do not discuss them here.

10. This claim is false; see chapter 4.

11. This utilitarian moral argument relies heavily on the truth of certain factual claims. Unless people do x (avoid meat/become vegetarians), y (irreversible environmental degradation) will result. Because y is morally undesirable (that is, causes suffering), people must do x to prevent or minimize y. Notice that y may occur even if people do x, but the claim is not usually intended to place all responsibility on each individual to prevent y alone but merely to do his or her part.

CHAPTER 2—ETHICAL VEGETARIANISM
AND TRADITIONAL MORAL THEORY

1. It is noteworthy that these same theories have been used in arguments against the moral requirement of vegetarianism. See, for instance, H. J. McCloskey (1979) and R. G. Frey (1983). Although these philosophers, whether arguing for or against moral vegetarianism, buttress their claims with appeals to rights or utility, close examination of their writings shows that their primary concern is whether nonhuman animals are morally considerable. Once their moral standing is established or ruled out, then each appeals to a moral theory of choice to delineate the exact nature of human duties to animals. Even excessively legalistic interpretations of rights theories rely on establishing the necessary and sufficient traits a being must have to belong to the moral community (see, for instance, Nicoll and Russell 1991). The brief review that follows here is not by any means meant as a comprehensive critique of animal rights or utilitarian animal welfare arguments. The debate *within* that tradition has generated a huge literature, review of which is not possible here. If I am correct, the tradition is self-defeating, and these internal arguments are not directly relevant to my thesis.

2. This method dates back at least to the Socratic dialogues of Plato. See, for instance, *Euthyphro*, in which Socrates asks the theologian for the essential characteristics of the virtue of piety: "show me what, precisely, this ideal is, so that, with my eye on it, and using it as a standard, I can say that any action done by you or anybody else is holy if it resembles this ideal, or, if it does not, can deny that it is holy" (Plato, *Euthyphro* 6e).

3. See Genesis 1:20–31; 9:1–3; Isaiah 1:11–15; 11:6-9; 66:3; Proverbs 12:1.

4. Singer's utilitarian moral theory actually does not permit adoption of rights for any being. Singer uses the term "rights" in his original edition (1975), but later retracts its usage in favor of "animal welfare" in order to remain consistent.

5. Singer (1975) states that the line of demarcation for which species of animals count is not clear (178–79).

6. Rollin's view is, in practice, more moderate than Regan's. Rollin has concentrated on practical concern for animal pain and animal consciousness, whereas Regan has campaigned for abolition of uses of animals in farming, research, education, and entertainment.

7. Bentham condemned the idea of individual "rights." No actions are intrinsically wrong. Conceivably, the rape of a child could be "right" in the proper situation; there is nothing *intrinsically wrong* about it, even if a "proper situation" could never arise. Even within traditional moral theory, utilitarianism has serious problems and is thought to be incommensurable with rights theory, which provides exactly the kind of immunities from the majority that utilitarianism cannot.

8. The general focus on interests, rather than on relationships and persons in contexts, is itself objectionable to many writers in feminist ethics. Plumwood briefly reviews the objections to focusing on interests and connects this focus to instrumentalism and division of the self (1991, esp. 18–22).

9. For a discussion of whether any rights can be thought to be absolute, see Vlastos (1962) and Feinberg (1973).

10. In traditional moral theory, the principle of equality is a separate principle that may or may not be used in the foundations of rights theory, but all major contemporary rights thinkers have assumed its validity or argued for it. See Vlastos (1962) and Feinberg (1973) for basic discussions; see also Rawls (1971).

11. Assume here also that others will be as happy or happier if the replacement is done.

12. There need not be a 1:1 relation here. Humans might have some essential nature and many ways of realizing or living in accord with it. Thus, many different interests might be consistently chosen by different people and still be "objectively good for the person." Often it is easier to understand conditions and situations that frustrate or corrupt one's interests than it is to list one or a set of ultimate goods for most or all people.

13. The inapplicability of moral theory to everyday moral dilemmas has been a topic of a great deal of discussion in the applied ethics literature. As John Kultgen (1998a) notes, "Unfortunately, attempts by philosophers to resolve practical issues of great concern to the public such as abortion, physician assisted suicide, our obligations to nature and future generations, and capital punishment have resulted in stalemates among members of the same schools of thought and more intractably among members of different schools" (325).

14. Alasdair MacIntyre's (1981) *After Virtue* has probably had the most influence in directing thought back to the virtues, although several other books and articles have been pivotal (Anscombe 1958; Foot 1978; Wallace 1978). MacIntyre argues that contemporary rule-based ethical theories are at an impasse and that moral debate has become endless and pointless.

15. Except see the remarks of Schneewind (1990) above.

16. Although MacIntyre (1981, 1984) and others writing in virtue ethics might disagree that an ethics of duty can support a virtue ethics, John Tomasi (1991) argues

that "because right holders must often decide whether to assert or withhold their claims, a rights-based system offers a ready framework for a system of ethics prescribing ideals to those right holders, ideals of what kinds of character are worth developing, of what kinds of persons they should be" (535).

17. My choice of the term "man" and the male pronoun is purposeful. Aristotle, as all his students know, did not think that women could be more than "natural slaves" and that the highest life was not open to them.

18. She cautions that this structure holds for Great Britain only with "important parallels and links with Germany and America." It would not be valid, she notes, for understanding the vegetarianism in India because there "vegetarianism and pollution are used to underwrite the elaborate social hierarchy of caste" whereas "in the west vegetarianism is strongly associated with an egalitarian, anti-structural ethic" (Twigg 1979, 15–16)

CHAPTER 3—FEMINISM AND
ETHICAL VEGETARIANISM

1. Elston (1987, 268–71, f. 47) notes that Queen Victoria gave private financial, but not public support to the cause of animals.

2. Donovan (1990) gives an extensive bibliography of the women writers who advocate either vegetarianism or animal welfare reform. See also Carol Adams (1990).

3. The turn-of-the-century impetus in England to vegetarianism cannot be separated from the antivivisectionist campaign, and both should be seen in the context of "a much wider public debate about sexual morality [and medicine] in the late nineteenth and early twentieth century. . . . The metaphor of medical science, and medical practice on women, as rape, became a dominant theme in antivivisection literature, especially that written by women, from the 1880s onwards. Women were explicitly invited to identify themselves with the animals, as potential victims of sexual assault by materialist medical men" (Elston 1987, 279). Elston reports on the women's opposition to compulsory vaccination laws that were enacted at the time and to ovariotomies done at great risk to women. Venereal diseases such as syphilis and gonorrhea caused great suffering, including dementia in syphilitics and blindness in newborns of women with gonorrhea. Many women contracted these diseases from their husbands' extramarital sexual encounters. These diseases remained incurable and without effective treatment until the development of antibiotics in the 1940s, although silver nitrate treatment of newborns' eyes to prevent blindness was discovered earlier. Several movements arose to fight for male chastity and continence. "Feminists involved with the Social Purity Union argued for women's right to control access to their own bodies in and outside of marriage, for celibacy as a normal way of living, free of male control, and, in some cases, for 'psychic love' as superior to mere carnality" (Elston 1987, 280). Social Darwinism was a hot topic of the day, and in 1897 Sarah Grand's best-selling *The Beth Book* has her heroine arguing against using vivisection to find cures for "'zymotic diseases' like measles or

smallpox, 'nature's way of ensuring the survival of the fittest'" (quoted in Elston 1987, 280). And Frances Power Cobbe, in a letter to *The Times* in 1888, suggested that "the demon of Whitechapel"—Jack the Ripper—could be "a physiologist delirious with cruelty" (cited in Elston 1987). These murders incited considerable consternation in the London population and "occasioned widespread concern about the dangers of unrestrained male sexuality in which doctors, especially vivisectors, figured strongly" (Elston 1987, 281; see also Walkowitz 1982).

4. For bibliographies of animal rights see Magel (1981, 1989); Friedman (1987); Gleason (1988); Christensen (1991); Feuerstein and Kheel (1991); Nordquist (1991).

5. Kohlberg's test for moral development is still given in colleges and universities, particularly in some colleges of education. Some women students report feeling frustrated and confused to find themselves scoring so low and begin to doubt even their moral character, despite the fact that they are often more truthful and far less violent than their male peers. Labeling such women "less morally well-developed" can have a devastating effect on their self-esteem and is unfair if what really matters for morality is not theory-structure but the actual actions and moral character of persons.

6. Here I adopt the notion of "fellow-feeling" as the meaning for sentiment, following Hume.

7. Although arguments that animals do not really feel pain seem incredible to ordinary persons, they had great persuasive power for scientists. Bernard Rollin (1989) gives a detailed history of what he calls "the common sense of science." As part of their training in scientific method, researchers, until very recently, were indoctrinated into an old behaviorist model of psychology that has its origins in the sixteenth century work of René Descartes and was elaborated in the early twentieth century by J. B. Watson when psychologists were concerned to make their science more "objective" by relying on observation of behavioral responses as opposed to "subjective" interpretations of action from the consciousness of animals and people. In the sixteenth century, one of the foundational beliefs about the nature of the universe was that human beings have an immortal soul and that all other things do not. Human beings, as the special creation of God, share this immortality with him. Descartes believed that the thinking, feeling mind was a separate substance that did not exist in space or time, just as God's existence is atemporal and nonextended. Descartes identified the mind and the soul, and since it was unthinkable that animals could have souls, he argued they could not have minds. And since the mind was the seat of all thought and sensation, then, animals could not experience pain. Although Newton would not articulate his physics for another half-century, mechanistic ideas about how the world worked were "in the air." Descartes and the Cartesians who followed him proposed that all bodies, whether human, animal, or physical, operated as machines. Machines may squeak and make noise, but they do not feel pain. The Cartesian legacy and its influence on human callousness in animal experimentation has been documented in nearly every modern argument for animal welfare and animal rights.

8. See Donovan (1992) for a review of various theoretical approaches to feminism.

9. Not all feminists endorsing care as an ethical foundation would agree that animals must be equally considerable (see, for instance, Noddings 1984).

10. Nothing anti-Boolean is implied by this claim: That is, a "logic" of domination is a pattern of behavior that flows from a certain kind of unethical or corrupt attitude. By changing the attitudes of the culture, the behavior will change, too, because a different "logic" will then obtain. Ecofeminists are apparently pointing to a psychosocial framework that governs most patterns of thought in our culture. A difficulty arises in that more than one attitude may cause the behavior (for example, domination) to occur, or the substitution of new attitudes may cause other unforeseen behaviors.

11. For example, both were featured at the Eighth Annual International Compassionate Living Festival, held in Raleigh, North Carolina, October 1–3, 1993, and the First National Conference for College Students and Teachers, "A New Generation for Animal Rights," held at Rutgers University-New Brunswick, New Jersey, July 29–August 1, 1993. Both conferences had prominent support from the Culture & Animals Foundation, whose founder and president is Tom Regan. Both conferences also featured other speakers arguing for animal rights from diverse, but sympathetic, theoretic and nontheoretic perspectives. Each featured vegan meals.

12. See, for instance, her reply to my arguments, based on the claim that someone who occasionally eats fish cannot be making valid arguments about the morality of vegetarianism (Adams 1995).

13. Curtin acknowledges that his view has many affinities with virtue ethics as well an ethic of care, and an ethic of capability to function, although he states that he finds the ethic of care view less helpful than he once did (1994, personal communication).

CHAPTER 4—A FEMINIST ARGUMENT
AGAINST ETHICAL VEGETARIANISM

1. Singer (1975) relies on the notion that "a vegetarian can expect to be at least as healthy as one who eats meat" (256). Unlike Regan, he does say that such health rests on the ability of the food industry to include supplements in our food. He also counsels pregnant women and other vulnerable groups to take extra care. But he does not notice the male bias in the vegan ideal (see 274–75).

2. That individuals actually carry different burdens in fulfilling their moral responsibilities is not always objectionable, however. For example, under traditional moral theory, all people are expected to keep their promises as a general rule. Some exceptions apply and rights or utilitarian theory can prescribe justifications for these exceptions, but the mere presence of a greater burden does not automatically grant an individual an exception to a valid moral rule. Many people will sometimes find it a greater burden than other people to keep a promise. Traditional moral theory would deny, however, that a valid moral rule or norm would systematically require self-sacrifices not required of others in circumstances beyond one's own control. So, a poor woman who buys a television set, promises to pay for it over time, and then finds she cannot make the payments does have more difficulty than a wealthy person in keeping her promise. But the rule is still impartial and nondiscriminatory if she chose to make the promise and could

have refrained from making it. Even though she belongs to a class that makes it more difficult to keep this particular promise, it does not thereby systematically foreclose her ability to make all promises without difficulty.

3. Dwyer is also Director of the Frances Stern Nutrition Center, New England Medical Center, Boston, Massachusetts.

4. In some areas of the world and for some subpopulations, breast-feeding is not recommended because certain disease pathogens pass through the milk and may infect the infant. HIV-positive women in the United States have been advised not to breast-feed (CDC 1985). The World Health Organization (WHO 1987) recommended that women in developing countries who are seropositive for HIV should continue breast-feeding because of its many advantages and uncertain risks. Hino (1989) has recommended that breast-feeding be discontinued in the Nagasaki Prefecture of Japan to halt the spread of HTLV-1, the retrovirus that causes adult T-cell leukemia (see also Institute of Medicine 1991, 170).

5. Vitamin B_{12} deficiency can be self-cured (or avoided) if one is willing to drink a strained extract of one's own feces. That unpalatable experiment was done in 1962 by Sheila Callender with vegan volunteers who were B_{12} deficient (cited in Herbert 1988, 852). She showed that colon bacteria of vegans make enough vitamin B_{12} to correct B_{12} deficiency but that B_{12} is not absorbed in the colon and is instead absorbed in the small bowel (Herbert 1988, 852). Reports of vitamin B_{12} in seaweed and spirulina show that these sources come in forms the body cannot use (Herbert 1988).

6. "Boiling milk destroys much of the vitamin B_{12} it provides, and such practices have been found to destroy much of the vitamin among some groups of very strict vegetarians who consumed small amounts of milk" (Dwyer 1991).

7. Smith (1990), reviewing the work of Henderson et al. (1987, 1990) reports that while vitamin D deficiency occurs only rarely in the United States, "in the UK, in contrast, late-onset rickets and osteomalacia made a dramatic reappearance with the immigration of Asians in the 1960s" (899). Osteomalacia disproportionately affects Asian women in the United Kingdom, and the studies of Henderson et al. (1990) found no significant association between exposure to daylight or wheat fiber intake and osteomalacia. But, in these women, the "presence of osteomalacia was strongly related to varying degrees of vegetarianism, being increased by the absence of eggs" (900). Finch et al. (1992) studied Asian vegetarians and non-vegetarians living in the United Kingdom and compared them with a control group of Europeans. They concluded that "those taking a vegetarian diet (in particular, Hindus) have an impaired seasonal rise in . . . vitamin D levels, and are at particular risk of metabolic bone disease" (509).

8. Calcium is also important in the regulation of blood pressure, and calcification of arteries may be seen in arteriosclerotic heart disease. Although ninety-nine percent of body calcium is deposited in the skeleton, the remaining one percent occurs in ionized form and circulates in blood and body tissues. Calcium ions participate in essential chemical functions, such as blood clotting, nerve transmission, muscle contraction and relaxation, membrane permeability, and enzyme activation (Johns Hopkins Medical Institutions 1994b, 4). "Having enough ionized calcium available for these

activities is so important that if the supply is inadequate, the body uses the skeleton as a bank from which it can withdraw calcium anytime it's necessary. But such withdrawals have a price: Over time they can lead to osteoporosis" (Johns Hopkins Medical Institutions, 4). Reducing dietary calcium has virtually no effect on the chemical functions affecting hypertension and heart disease: "While calcium ions help regulate blood pressure . . . , the number of calcium ions in the body remains relatively constant regardless of diet" (4). So eating less calcium-rich foods will not lower hypertension or slow the buildup of calcium that occurs in arteriosclerosis (4).

9. The economic cost is also very high: "Annual direct medical costs of osteoporosis incurred by American women aged 45 and older are estimated at $5.2 billion in 1986" (Phillips *et al.* 1988). This estimate is now over a decade old; with the rate of inflation of medical costs in the past decade, the actual cost may now be double or triple that figure.

10. At least one new drug has been developed to increase bone in older people, however.

11. In 1991, Hernandez-Avila *et al.* reported increased risk of hip fracture in women who consumed greater amounts of caffeine compared with those women who drank little or none; however, Barrett-Connor *et al.* (1994) did a long-term study of almost one thousand women and report that a lifetime of coffee drinking can be counteracted by drinking as little as one glass of milk per day. Moderate alcohol intake was associated with increased risk of both hip and forearm fractures (Hernandez-Avila *et al.* 1991). Weight-bearing physical exercise can have a positive effect on bone density and may slow down bone loss in postmenopausal women (Johns Hopkins Medical Institutions 1994a).

12. Inherited factors also determine bone mass as confirmed by studies of mother-daughter pairs and twins (Pocock *et al.* 1987; Pollitzer and Anderson 1989; Lutz and Tesar 1990). And Morrison *et al.* (1994) have reported the discovery of a gene for at least one type of osteoporosis (see also Mundy 1994).

13. Many people—up to seventy percent of the world's population—are lactose intolerant, although commercial products are available in western countries to abate the problem; see Peikin (1991). Persistent lactase activity, or the ability to digest milk past childhood, is governed by a gene that occurs in populations in Europe and Africa with a long history of dairy farming (National Research Council 1989a). Most adults who are genetically lactose intolerant can tolerate 250 milliliters of milk per day, and yogurt, cheeses, and other dairy products are better tolerated (National Research Council 1989a).

14. Risk was greatest for cancers of the esophagus, bladder, and to a lesser extent of the colon and lung (data adjusted for age and smoking habits).

15. Differentiation is the process that occurs during development and in the normal course of regeneration. Differentiation makes a cell the kind of cell it is and results in its having a specific function, such as being a skin cell, brain cell, liver cell, heart muscle cell, blood cell, and so forth. In differentiated cells, only part of the genetic material is active or "turned on."

16. These figures are improvements over the life expectancy of 44.7 years for females and 46.4 years for males cited in Soysa (1987) from U.N. Demographic Year-book for 1978. Presumably, improvements in the food supply and medical care have permitted lengthening the life span, and the pattern of women living longer than men in industrialized countries may now be exemplified in India as well. Whether these figures account for disproportionate mortality among females under the age of adolescence is unknown.

17. In December 1992, the Institute of Medicine's Food and Nutrition Board sponsored the symposium "Nutrition and Minority Health: The Interplay of Food, Culture, Genetics, and Environment" devoted to discussion of these issues.

18. The RDA for children under eleven is 800 mg of calcium per day (Ca/day), for adolescents and young adults age 11–24 is 1200 mg Ca/day, and for adults twenty-five and over is 800 mg Ca/day. Bourgoin et al. (1993) discovered that the average micrograms of lead per 800 mg of calcium was: bonemeal 11.33 µg; "natural source" (oyster shell) carbonate 6.05 µg; dolomite 4.17 µg; chelates 1.64 µg; laboratory-made "refined" carbonate 0.92 µg; by contrast, milk contained 0.71 µg (Table 3, 1157; see also Liebman 1993).

19. Vegans would be unlikely to take bonemeal or oyster shell supplements, which means they would have to take dolomite or "refined" supplements and even these may deliver several times the dose of lead that milk does.

20. The recent discovery that women whose levels of folic acid were low before they became pregnant increases the likelihood of birth defects points in this direction (Tufts University 1994a). As an aside, there is considerable debate about whether folic acid supplements should be used since these can mask other conditions, such as pernicious anemia (vitamin B_{12} deficiency). Good sources of folic acid are dark green leafy vegetables, citrus fruits and juice, yeast, bread, and fortified cereals. "But a woman would have to eat, for example, more than a cup of cooked broccoli, two-thirds of a cup of cooked spinach, and about a cup of cooked turnip greens each day to obtain the 0.4 milligram of the nutrient government officials recommend. Most women typically consume foods that provide only about half that amount" (Tufts University 1994a, 1). Diets that increase vegetable consumption are certainly warranted.

21. It is a common but incorrect assumption that vegetarian diets must be low in fat and meat-containing diets must be high in fat, but vegans who eat too many fried foods (such as french fried potatoes), margarine, nut butters, and other fatty plant foods may easily exceed the limit on daily fat intake recommended for heart safety. Soy products are usually a staple of a vegan diet, but their fat content is much higher than skim dairy products. For example, one cup of soy milk contains 184 kcal, 6.2 g fat, 11.9 g protein, and 1.2 mg elemental calcium, or about twice the calories, 14 times the fat, 130 percent of the protein, and 4.3 percent of the calcium of the same amount of skim milk (86 kcal, .44 g fat, 8.35 g protein, 28 mg calcium). Three cups of skim milk contribute only 1.32 g/fat. Tofu is a compact source of protein, but it is also a compact source of fat since over half its calories come from fat (Robertson *et al.* 1986). Semivegetarian diets, low in unsaturated fat and cholesterol, may be planned that include some meat.

22. Barrett-Connor and Bush (1991) report that "most, but not all, studies of hormone replacement therapy in postmenopausal women show around a fifty percent reduction in risk of a coronary event in women using unopposed oral estrogen" (1861).

23. In 1992, the National Institutes of Health funded a "study of more than 60,000 postmenopausal women . . . to answer questions about the effect of diet and estrogen replacement therapy on cardiovascular health and the prevention of breast cancer and osteoporosis" (Holloway and Yam 1992, 18).

24. Federal agencies such as U.S. Department of Agriculture and U.S. Department of Health and Welfare also have ignored differences in ethnicity in their recommendations for diet. See, for example, Perkin and McCann (1984).

25. Although ethics has presupposed this kind of ideal, it does not seem necessary that science do so except as a practical stratagem applied to individual experiments. Indeed, it seems a consequence of scientific method that more and more individual differences rather than similarities will be delineated. Considerations of space do not permit defense of that claim here, although I hope to make it a future project.

26. Singer's view is less absolute than Regan's because Singer is a utilitarian. If it could be shown that more aggregate harm would result from universal vegan diets, then he could admit some use of animal products and even some meat eating. His view still fails on the same assumptions as Regan's (see chapter 2).

27. Westernized education does not assure knowledge about food and nutrition. For instance, a highly educated group of people formed a primarily vegan commune known as The Farm in Summertown, Tennessee, in the late 1960s. Despite their education, they apparently were not nutritionally aware of the risks associated with veganism. In 1971, the Public Health Service examined and treated several of the women and children for vitamin B_{12}, iron, and possible protein deficiencies. Subsequently, the community became very interested in monitoring the nutritional health of its members. The Farm established its research organization ETHOS and a health clinic to monitor the growth of the children and health of the community. Members began taking vitamin B_{12}, iron, and calcium supplements after 1971. Although children on The Farm are typically somewhat shorter in stature and lighter in weight than all or part of the U.S. population, they are otherwise healthy (Carter *et al.* 1987; O'Connell *et al.* 1989). This shows that even in Western countries, special nutritional education and medical care are advisable for those on vegan diets. Dwyer (1991) advises gestating and lactating vegan women, vegan infants, and elderly vegans to obtain nutritional counseling and carefully plan their diets before attempting to eliminate meat, fish, milk, and eggs from their diets. Continued reports of nutritional deficiencies among vegan women and children that appear in the literature offer good reasons to take the "careful planning" requirement seriously (Dagnelie *et al.* 1989, 1990; Doyle *et al.* 1989). Patricia Mutch (1988) has reviewed the practical uses of food guides developed by nutritionists and finds that, although all of them have problems, their use combined with general guidelines would be much more satisfactory in achieving nutritional adequacy than using general guidelines alone.

28. For example, from 75–100 different languages are spoken in the Los Angeles schools; parents of these children do not speak English (Meyer 1992; Taliaferro and

Murr 1991). About twenty-four different languages are spoken by children in the school district in my own small town of 18,000.

29. See also Wolf (1991), Chapkis (1986), Galler (1984), Morgan (1991), and Walker (1983) for discussions of the connections of beauty to female goodness.

30. Brownell is Co-Director of the Yale Center for Eating and Weight Disorders.

31. Barlow and Durand (1995) define "anorexia nervosa [as] a person's refusal to eat anything except minimal amounts of food, with the result that body weight sometimes drops to dangerously low levels. In bulimia nervosa, attempts to restrict food intake result in out-of-control eating episodes, or binges, often followed by self-induced vomiting, excessive use of laxatives, or other attempts to 'purge' (get rid of) the food just eaten" (299).

32. Although whole foods offer the best nutrition, some areas of the world simply cannot grow or tolerate the introduction of these foods grown locally. The introduction of cattle to Africa has accelerated desertification, and monocropped, chemical and mechanized agriculture has disenfranchised millions of peasants around the world (Lappé 1982). Some conditions of deficiency have been brought about by Westernization, but it would be a mistake to assume that traditional recipes are automatically balanced to cope with long-term vegan requirements. Space limitations preclude further documentation and discussion of these important concerns.

33. Joan Dye Gussow (1994) argues that agricultural sustainability requires continuation of animal production, although at a much lower level. Her holistic outlook generally accords with that of Frances Moore Lappé (1982), who had originally argued for vegetarianism on ecological grounds in her 1971 edition of *Diet for a Small Planet* and later proposed a modified position in her tenth edition (1982). See also Lewis (1994) for a brief recap of the ecological argument against meat consumption.

CHAPTER 5—BIAS, REASONING, AND SCIENTIFIC STUDIES

1. An ethical vegetarian could still claim that she and others have a moral obligation to continue the practice. One possible ground would be pacificism based on faith that such a commitment is right no matter what the facts may be. The question of whether such a ground is adequate is discussed in chapter 1.

2. Bollet (1992) reports that over three million cases and 100,000 deaths occurred in an epidemic of pellagra (multivitamin deficiency usually treated with niacin supplementation) in fifteen southern states of the United States from about 1906 to 1940. "In the late nineteenth century, beriberi (vitamin B_1 deficiency) was prevalent in Japan, the Dutch East Indies (Indonesia), the Philippines, Brazil, and other countries where rice was the staple food" (Yokoi and Sandstead 1992). Enrichment of flours and grains by adding back B–vitamins after milling has eliminated these deficiencies in industrialized countries. "Rickets plagued the children who lived in the industrial cities of North America and Europe from the seventeenth through the nineteenth century. At

the beginning of this century, over 85 percent of the children living in these areas had rickets" (Holick *et al.* 1992, 1178). Lebrun *et al.* (1993) report that rickets has largely disappeared in Canada, but still frequently occurs in a few areas with primarily native populations. Vitamin D fortification of milk began shortly after the method was discovered in 1924, and rickets thereafter subsided as a major public health problem in Europe and North America (Holick *et al.* 1992).

3. "The incidence of iron deficiency anemia, rickets, and zinc deficiency is very high in Chinese preschool children" (Chen *et al.* 1992; see also Kantha 1990). Zhao (1992) also reports that riboflavin, zinc, and calcium intakes are inadequate in many Beijing, China, adults and elderly. Zhu (1990) reports on 2,041 cases of osteoporosis in China. "In Indonesia beriberi is still endemic" (Djoenaidi *et al.* 1992). Sharma and Sharma (1992) report iron deficiency anemia, pellagra, and vitamin A deficiency in pregnant tribal women in India. Schnitzler *et al.* (1994) report calcium deficiency, rickets and osteomalacia among Black African teenagers in South Africa who come from areas where calcium consumption is low and dairy products are unavailable.

4. When absorption is considered, 20 percent of the iron from lean beef is absorbable and 18 percent from chicken compared to 7 percent from soybeans, 1.6 percent from black beans, 1.4 percent from spinach, and 4.4 percent from lettuce (Scrimshaw 1991, graph, 48). This means that the adolescent in the example would be required to eat 12 times as much spinach as given in the example (9 cups) and 4.5 times as much lettuce (18 cups) to get the same iron as in the beef patty.

5. On September 29, 1992, the American Academy of Pediatrics (AAP 1992) issued a response to the claims of Physicians Committee for Responsible Medicine (PCRM 1991) that milk and other dairy products were no longer needed for children's health. While the AAP recommended that only breast milk or iron-fortified infant formula be used in the first year of life, they affirm the value of milk as a nutritional source in childhood. Since 1976, AAP has advised that skim milk not be given in the first two years of life because infants need more calories than skim milk can provide; whole or perhaps two percent milk (if the physician recommends it) may be given after one year. The AAP affirms that "milk is a major source of nutrition" and that "the Academy will not be altering its recommendation that milk be a standard part of children's diets" (1992, 30).

6. Despite the current judgment of nutritionists that lifelong adequate calcium intake is essential to prevention of osteoporosis, philosophers and other lay critics sometimes claim that researchers are misconstruing the causal relationship (Pluhar 1993, Varner 1994a). Their complaint runs roughly like this: People in Western nations use many more dairy products than people in other parts of the world; they also have the highest incidence of osteoporosis. Their high calcium and high protein consumption is the cause of this disease, and if people in affluent countries used fewer dairy products the rate of osteoporosis would decline. These critics usually cite Hegsted (1986), who proposed a complex theory based on this correlation. Although correlations provide important research clues, correlations are not causes; they are two events that occur together. Countries with the highest consumption of dairy products also have the

largest populations of older people, in whom osteoporosis is most prevalent. So, correlations exist for consuming dairy products, living a long life, and getting osteoporosis. On the correlation of high protein and osteoporosis, Dwyer and Loew (1994) point out: "Vegan diets are not necessarily lower in protein than other diets, so altered calcium excretion due to lower protein intakes cannot be assumed" (101). Further, "the belief that those who do not use milk and milk products have lower calcium needs is not correct" (94). Osteoporosis is seen in younger women in countries where calcium intakes are very low (Pollitzer and Anderson 1989; Nordin 1966). Neil Barnard (1989) of PCRM and John Robbins (*Diet for a New America*, 1987) claim that it is specifically animal protein that causes osteoporosis and not plant protein. What about that? Here we have a distortion of what turns out to be old data from 1981. Schardt (1993) reviews their claims and the more recent nutritional evidence on animal protein and osteoporosis, kidney disease, heart disease, and cancer. He interviewed Mark Hegsted, a well-known researcher on the link between osteoporosis and calcium, whose 1986 hypothesis is mentioned above (Hegsted 1986) and is often cited by PCRM and its supporters (PCRM 1991; Varner 1994; Pluhar 1992). Hegsted acknowledges that the countries with the highest rates of osteoporosis also consume the most protein and calcium: "But that doesn't mean the protein and calcium are causing the osteoporosis. . . . It could be something else in their diet or lifestyle" (7). Schardt interviews several other nutrition researchers and explains that "the amount of calcium you lose [from eating high amounts of protein] isn't as great as researchers once thought" (1993). And in a commentary, Spencer *et al.* (1988) review the question of whether protein and phosphorus cause calcium loss. They note that these are misconceptions that can do harm and that while experiments with purified protein did cause calcium loss, "studies with adults suggest that high protein *foods* do not cause calcium loss" (emphasis added, 657).

7. The Dutch Kushi macrobiotic families studied by Dagnelie *et al.* (1989, 1990) illustrate this point well. The persistence of slow growth and deficiencies in infants and children of these families prompted Dagnelie *et al.* to recommend a dietary change, and Kushi directed the followers to change the diet to include some fish, but many followers have refused. Their children remain deficient.

8. The term "blind" here is a technical term; it should be viewed in the positive sense of enabling the scientist to discover something apart from her own personal interests, goals, and prejudices. I apologize to anyone who finds any metaphorical use of the term offensive, but alternative terms are not available.

9. "A study is *blind* if the subjects cannot tell whether they are in the experimental or control group. . . . A study is called *double-blind* if the experimenters making the diagnosis are also kept in the dark about which subjects are in which group" (Giere 1991, 253–54). Subjects in the control group are typically given placebos (pills or procedures to match what is done to the experimental group) so that in every outward way each group is treated the same. Studies should be randomized. The study group is chosen from a random sample of the whole population of interest, and the sample members are, in turn, randomly assigned to the experimental group or to the control group (Giere 1991, 227). Randomization to each group is so standard that it is sometimes

assumed in reports and may not be mentioned. It is usually reasonable to assume random assignment to one group or the other, but it is always important to look for a control group.

Giere (1991) goes on to explain that prospective and retrospective studies cannot be completely randomized. Instead, prospective studies look at populations that exhibit a suspected *cause* (such as smoking) of an effect (such as cancer). Retrospective studies are done on populations that exhibit the *effect* already. In a *prospective* study, because the population is picked out for study based on a particular cause, the group cannot be chosen at random (for example, smokers only are picked). The researcher can still randomize among the group by assignments to control or experimental group, however. In a good prospective study, a second, matched group is chosen (for instance, nonsmokers) so that the "two groups . . . are, on average, similar in every feature *except* the expected causal factor" (Giere 1991, 237). So, if researchers want to know whether smoking causes lung cancer, only smokers with no signs or symptoms would be included in the study. The two groups are followed over time to see whether those in the group with the suspected cause develop significantly more cases of the effect (lung cancer) than those who do not exhibit the cause. These studies are called "prospective" because they look to the future and the effect occurs later in time. A *retrospective* study "begins with a sample of subjects that already have the *effect* . . . and attempts to look back in time to discover the *cause*. . . . Random sampling plays almost no role in retrospective studies" (Giere 1991, 245). A "control group is still chosen to match the subjects in the experimental group for other variables that might be causally relevant" (246). With prospective and retrospective studies, the self-selection present in the experimental group may bias the study (Giere 1991, 247). Retrospective studies have the further defect that the experimental group itself is not at all a random sample—the subjects "get into the experimental group because something special has happened to them" (248). Retrospective studies cannot estimate "the percentage of the population that would or would not get the *effect* depending on whether they all had the *cause*" (248). Giere (1991) notes that retrospective studies offer "limited usefulness in decision making" and other more reliable information must be used in conjunction with them (249).

10. This is the reason I have had my scientific claims in nutrition read and assessed for accuracy by three different nutritionists.

11. Giere (1991) gives the example that lung cancer is highly correlated with the use of ashtrays; if correlation were as good as cause, one could conclude that ashtray use causes lung cancer. But it is the third factor interacting with these—smoking—that is the real cause of lung cancer. Incidentally, these analogies are meant to illustrate logical concepts concerning causality and should not be construed to be commenting on vegetarianism. I have purposely chosen other examples to avoid false implications of posited causal connections.

12. Absolute certainty is not possible in inductive or scientific reasoning about events in the world. It is always possible that we will find some evidence that dashes the best warranted beliefs. To paraphrase David Hume, we have no certainty that sun will rise tomorrow. We might find out it will supernova instead. But, of course, if induction

is a valid principle of reason, then we are well-warranted in believing that it will rise. It would be irrational to believe that it will not, given all the evidence we have to believe that it will.

13. Breast milk is preferred for infants, with iron supplementation coming in cereals after six months and in vitamin drops. But some women cannot or do not breast feed.

14. And I might add that when I published my arguments, ethical vegans were the first to point out my "immorality" to me and to others, thereby leading me again to infer that they regarded themselves as morally superior for what they eat or do not eat.

15. Blood transfusions were not considered dangerous in 1976, but by 1983 an untested blood supply accounted for several cases of HIV infection. I simply chose the most conservative measure first.

16. Some authors refer to this as the "naturalistic fallacy." Philosophers often reserve this latter name for the fallacy ascribed to G. E. Moore in positing a "non-natural property" in things, events, or actions perceived as "good."

CHAPTER 6—GENDER EQUALITY
AND INTERSPECIES EQUALITY

1. For a discussion of the many ways the female body has been constructed as inferior or lacking in comparison to the male in Western culture, see Nancy Tuana, *The Less Noble Sex: Scientific, Religious, and Philosophical Conceptions of Woman's Nature* (1993). Tuana points out that such conceptions permeate our culture even today in ways that may be opaque to our understanding.

2. Adams herself *claims* to embrace a feminist rather than a traditionalist moral framework. I simply point out that her use of the language of rights, her absolutist reliance on rules, and the structure of her arguments are hallmarks of traditional rights theory.

3. The assimilationist attitude was pervasive at the time preceding the foregoing Supreme Court decision and extended to nonactionable cases as well. For example, when I was a young working mother in the 1970s, it was assumed that if I wished to be considered an equal with most male workers I would not take a single day off during my pregnancy or later to care for my sick child. In fact, most women who were well-regarded by their male supervisors and whose jobs were most secure were those who took no sick leave to care for children.

4. For example, both Regan and Frey appeared together on the program at the Biotechnology Institute, Iowa State University, Ames, May 18, 1993, where each acknowledged the many appearances they had done together.

5. The Center for Science in the Public Interest (1994) reports that "since 1986, more than 110,000 children have been poisoned by iron supplements or iron-containing multivitamins. More than thirty have died, some after swallowing as few as *five* tablets" (3, italics in original).

6. For example, see works by Jean-Paul Sartre, Martin Heidegger, and other existentialists.

CHAPTER 7—FEMINIST
AESTHETIC SEMIVEGETARIANISM

1. Carol Adams and other feminist vegetarians such as Josephine Donovan, Greta Gaard, and Lori Gruen would also use the language of alienation, subject-object dichotomies, and rejection of domination and patriarchy as part of the reasons to reject meat eating. However, their views are absolutist in nature and rely on the structure of traditional moral theory rather than feminist contextualism (see chapter 3).

2. I do not believe the medicalization of morality is generally defensible. Using "healthy" or "unhealthy" in place of "good" or "bad" tends to discourage responsibility by removing the concepts of will, decision making, and choice. People are usually not held responsible for their illnesses. But we are responsible for our choices. Eliding the distinction between morality and illness creates confusion about when we ought to hold others responsible.

3. Deane Curtin does not intend that his view is a form of egoism or even ethical egoism. I am pointing out that it collapses to that because of logical inconsistencies in the ethical framework he adopts.

4. Curtin is *not* intending to endorse selfishness. I merely argue that his view unfortunately sounds good but collapses to doing whatever one wants. As long as one wants the peace and nonviolence Curtin proposes, then all is well. But what of those who practice violence and exploitation? Moral arguments must go beyond preaching to the choir.

5. Notice, too, the parallels to the idea of the "noble savage" in Rousseau and the view of human nature expressed in Marx and Engels—that of a pure human being deformed by an artificial society.

6. Anyone who has read Carol Adams' work cannot fail to see in her linguistic constructions the parallel reasoning and word-for-word, chapter-and-verse recitation of the century or older ideology described by Twigg (1979).

7. A sad example of this is Adele Davis (1954), one of the earliest advocates of diet as a preventative of illness. It was particularly poignant when she died of cancer in 1974.

8. Some interesting ideas come to mind here. In a semivegetarian society, would it be right for steakhouses to exist? Well, such places do promote heavy meat eating. Right now, it's excessive. But suppose that in a semivegetarian society, people only frequented such places for celebratory events and ate little or no meat at other times?

9. My supposition here does not imply that infants *are* moral agents; but parents must be guided by what they believe is in the child's best interest and so they must decide what kind of diet they should feed their children.

10. Pancreatic implantation of insulin-producing cells for cure of diabetes could be considered as a hypothetical example, although to be more analogous we should assume the surgery has gone beyond the experimental stage.

11. This example also illustrates something else about the presumed norm in traditionalist ethical vegetarianism (that is, Adams, Donovan, Gaard, Gruen, Regan, Singer, Varner): The ideal person has no one else dependent upon him and for whom he must make decisions and no one else's interests to protect but his own. He is not a parent.

References

Acosta, Phyllis B. 1988. Availability of essential amino acids and nitrogen in vegan diets. *American Journal of Clinical Nutrition* 48: 868–74.

Adams, Carol J. 1975. The Oedible complex: Feminism and vegetarianism. In Gina Covina and Laurel Galana, eds., *The Lesbian Reader*. Oakland, Calif.: Amazon.

———. 1976. Vegetarianism: The inedible complex. *Second Wave* 4 (4): 36–42.

———. 1990. *The Sexual Politics of Meat: A Feminist-Vegetarian Critical Theory*. New York: Continuum.

———. 1991. Ecofeminism and the eating of animals. *Hypatia* 6:1 (Spring): 125–45.

———. 1993. The feminist traffic in animals. In Greta Gaard, ed., *Ecofeminism: Women, Animals, Nature*, 195–218. Philadelphia: Temple University Press.

———. 1994. *Neither Man Nor Beast: Feminism and the Defense of Animals*. New York: Continuum.

———. 1995. Comment on George's "Should Feminists Be Vegetarians?" *Signs* 21:1 (Autumn): 221–25.

Alcoff, Linda, and Elizabeth Potter, eds. 1993. *Feminist Epistemologies*. New York: Routledge.

Allen, Lindsay H. 1986. Calcium and osteoporosis. *Nutrition Today* 21 (May/June): 6–10.

Allen, Paula Gunn. 1986. *The Sacred Hoop: Recovering the Feminine in American Indian Traditions*. Boston: Beacon.

American Academy of Pediatrics. 1992. Media alert: AAP responds to PCRM statement on milk consumption. Chicago, September 29. *American Academy of Pediatrics*, 141 Northwest Point Blvd., Elk Grove Village, Ill.

Ames, Katherine, Mary Hager, Larry Wilson, and Linda Buckley. 1990. Our bodies, our selves: A bias against women in health research. *Newsweek* (December 17): 60.

Anderson, Jackie. 1994. Separatism, feminism, and the betrayal of reform. *Signs* 19:2 (Winter): 437–448.

Anonymous. 1979. Vitamin B_{12} deficiency in the breast-fed infant of a strict vegetarian. *Nutrition Reviews* 37: 142–44.

Anscombe, G. E. M. 1958. Modern moral philosophy. Reprinted in her *Ethics, Religion and Politics*, Collected Philosophical Papers, vol. 3, 26–42. Minneapolis: University of Minnesota Press, 1981.

Aristotle. 1984. *Nichomachean Ethics*. In Jonathan Barnes, ed., *The Complete Works of Aristotle*, revised Oxford translation. Princeton, N. J.: Princeton University Press.

Auchmutey, Jim. 1986. Animal crackers: The animal-rights movement is a comical tragedy that's probably playing at a campus near you. *Campus Voice* (Winter): 42–47.

Bakan, R., C. L. Birmingham, L. Aeberhardt, and E. M. Goldner. 1993. Dietary zinc intake of vegetarian and nonvegetarian patients with anorexia nervosa. *International Journal of Eating Disorders* 13:2 (March): 229–33.

Bardare, M., G. Magnolfi, and G. Zoni. 1988. Soy sensitivity: Personal observations on 71 children with food intolerance. *Allergie et Immunologie* 20: 63–68.

Barlow, David H., and V. Mark Durand. 1995. Eating disorders. In *Abnormal Psychology: An Integrative Approach*, Chapter 8. Pacific Grove, Calif.: Brooks/Cole Publishing Co.

Barnard, Neil. 1989. Beyond the myths about osteoporosis. *The Animals' Agenda* (November): 7.

Barrett-Connor, E., and T. L. Bush. 1991. Estrogen and coronary heart disease in women. *Journal of the American Medical Association* 265:14 (April 10): 1861–67.

Barrett-Connor, E., J. C. Chang, and S. L. Edelstein. 1994. Coffee-associated osteoporosis offset by daily milk consumption: The Rancho Bernardo study. *Journal of the American Medical Association* 271:4 (January 26): 280–83.

Beardsworth, Alan, and Teresa Keil. 1991. Health-related beliefs and dietary practices among vegetarians and vegans: A qualitative study. *Health Education Journal* 50(1): 38–42.

Begley, Sharon. 1990. These rats die for our sins. *Newsweek* (October 22): 68.

Belasco, Warren J. 1989. *Appetite for Change: How the Counterculture Took on the Food Industry, 1966–1988*. New York: Pantheon Books.

Bell, Linda A., ed. 1983. *Visions of Women*. Clifton, N.J.: Humana Press.

Bell, Rudolph M. 1985. *Holy Anorexia*. Chicago: University of Chicago Press.

Bentham, Jeremy. (1789) 1974. *Introduction to the Principles of Morals and Legislation*. Chap. I–IV. Reprinted in Mary Warnock, ed., *John Stuart Mill: Utilitarianism, On Liberty, Essay on Bentham Together with Selected Writings of Jeremy Bentham and John Austin*. New York: New American Library, Inc., 1962.

Bollet, Alfred Jay. 1992. Politics and pellagra: The epidemic of pellagra in the U.S. in the early twentieth century. *Yale Journal of Biology and Medicine* 65: 211–221.

Bothwell, T. H., R. D. Baynes, B. J. MacFarlane, and A. P. MacPhail. 1989. Nutritional iron requirements and food iron absorption. *Journal of Internal Medicine* 226: 357–65.

Bourgoin, Bernard P., Douglas R. Evans, Jack R. Cornett, Susanne M. Lingard, and Alfredo J. Quattrone. 1993. Lead content in 70 brands of dietary calcium supplements. *American Journal of Public Health* 83 (August): 1155–60.

Bowker, John. 1986. Introduction: Religions and the rights of animals. In Tom Regan, ed., *Animal Sacrifices: Religious Perspectives on the Use of Animals in Science*, 3–14. Philadelphia: Temple University Press.

Brotman, Andrew W. 1994. What works in the treatment of anorexia nervosa? *Harvard Mental Health Letter* 10:7 (January): 8.

Brownell, Kelly D. 1998. "Oh, you beautiful (unrealistic) doll." http://southbound. com.my/souths/cap/title/oh.htm (October 24).

———, and C. G. Fairburn, eds. 1995. *Eating Disorders and Obesity: A Comprehensive Handbook.* N.Y.: Guilford.

Brumberg, Joan Jacobs. 1988. *Fasting Girls: The Emergence of Anorexia Nervosa as a Modern Disease.* Cambridge: Harvard University Press.

Bull-McDonough, Andrea. 1993. Eating disorders. In Patricia M. Queen and Carol E. Lang, eds., *Handbook of Pediatric Nutrition.* Gaithersburg, Md.: Aspen Publishers.

Bynum, Caroline Walker. 1987. *Holy Feast and Holy Fast.* Berkeley and Los Angeles: University of California Press.

Calkins, Beverly M. 1988. Executive summary of the Congress [on Vegetarian Nutrition]. *American Journal of Clinical Nutrition* 48:3 (September): 709–711.

Campbell, T. Colin, Chen Junshi, Thierry Brun, Banoo Parpia, Qu Yinsheng, Chen Chumming, and Catherine Geissler. 1992. China: From diseases of poverty to diseases of affluence. Policy implications of the epidemiological transition. *Ecology of Food and Nutrition* 27: 133–44.

Campbell, T. Colin, Junshi Chen, Chongbo Liu, Junyao Li, and Banoo Parpia. 1990a. Non-association of aflatoxin with primary liver cancer in a cross-sectional ecological survey in the People's Republic of China. *Cancer Research* 50 (November 1): 6882–93.

Campbell, T. Colin, Thierry Brun, Junshi Chen, F. Zulin, and Banoo Parpia. 1990b. Questioning riboflavin recommendations on the basis of a survey in China. *American Journal of Clinical Nutrition* 51: 436–45.

Campbell-Brown, M., R. J. Ward, A. P. Haines, W. R. S. North, R. Abraham, I. R. McFadyen, J. R. Turnlund, and J. C. King. 1985. Zinc and copper in Asian pregnancies—Is there evidence for a nutritional deficiency? *British Journal of Obstetrics and Gynecology* 92 (September): 875-85.

Card, Claudia. 1990. Caring and evil. *Hypatia* 5:1 (Spring): 101–8.

Carrillo Díaz, Teresa, Manuela Cuevas Agustin, M. Luz Díez Gómez, Eloy Losada Cosme, and Ignacio Moneo Goiri. 1986. Diagnóstico immunológico *in vitro* en la hipersensibilidad a legumbres. [In vitro immunologic diagnosis of hypersensitivity to legumes]. *Allergologia et Immunopathologia* 14(2): 139–46.

Carson, Gerald. 1957. *Cornflake Crusade.* New York: Rinehart.

Carter, James P., Tami Furman, and H. Robert Hutcheson. 1987. Preeclampsia and reproductive performance in a community of vegans. *Southern Medical Journal* 80:6 (June): 692–7.

Centers for Disease Control (CDC). 1985. Recommendations for assisting in the prevention of perinatal transmission of human T-lymphotropic virus type III/lymphadenopathy-associated virus and acquired immunodeficiency syndrome. *Morbidity and Mortality Weekly Report* 34: 721–32.

Center for Science in the Public Interest. 1994. Iron-clad containers. *Nutrition Action Health Letter* 21:10 (December): 3.

Chapkis, Wendy. 1986. *Beauty Secrets.* Boston: South End Press.

Chen, Junshi, T. Colin Campbell, Li Junyao, and Richard Peto. 1990. *Diet, Life-Style, and Mortality in China.* Oxford: Oxford University Press.

Chen Xue-Cun, Wen-Guang Wang, Huai-Cheng Yan, Tai-an Yin, and Qing-Mei Xu. 1992. Studies on iron deficiency anemia, rickets and zinc deficiency and their prevention among Chinese preschool children. *Progress in Food and Nutrition Science* 16: 263–77.

Christensen, John O. 1991. *Animal Experimentation, Animal Rights: A Bibliography of Recent References.* Monticello, Ill.: Vance Bibliographies.

Cimoch, Paul J. (M.D.) 1993. Treating wasting and malnutrition in HIV/AIDS patients. *Nutrition & the M.D.* 19:9 (September): 1–4.

Clemens, T. L., S. L. Henderson, J. S. Adams, and M.F. Holick. 1982. Increased skin pigment reduces capacity of skin to synthesize vitamin D_3. *Lancet* 1: 74–6.

Clutton-Brock, Juliet. 1987. *A Natural History of Domesticated Mammals.* Austin: University of Texas Press.

Collard, Andrée, with Joyce Contrucci. 1989. *Rape of the Wild: Man's Violence Against Animals and the Earth.* Bloomington: Indiana University Press.

Copi, Irving M., and Carl Cohen. 1990. *Introduction to Logic.* 8th ed. New York: Macmillan.

Council on Scientific Affairs, American Medical Association. 1987. Vitamin preparations as dietary supplements and as therapeutic agents. *Journal of the American Medical Association* 257:14 (April 10): 1929–36.

Cowley, Geoffrey with Mary Hager, Lisa Drew, Tessa Namuth, Lynda Wright, Andrew Murr, Nonny Abbott, and Kate Robins. 1988. The battle over animal rights: A question of suffering and science, of pain and progress. *Newsweek* (December 26): 50–59.

Curtin, Deane W. 1992a. Food/body/person. In Deane W. Curtin and Lisa M. Heldke, eds., *Cooking, Eating, Thinking: Transformative Philosophies of Food,* 3–22. Bloomington: Indiana University Press.

———. 1992b. Recipes for values. In Deane W. Curtin and Lisa M. Heldke, eds., *Cooking, Eating, Thinking: Transformative Philosophies of Food,* 123–44. Bloomington: Indiana University Press.

———. 1991. Toward an ecological ethic of care. *Hypatia* 6:1 (Spring): 60–74.

Dagnelie, Pieter C., Wija A. van Staveren, Freddy J.V.R.A. Vergote, Pieter G. Dingjan, Henk van den Berg, and Joseph G.A.J. Hautvast. 1989. Increased risk of vitamin B_{12} and iron deficiency in infants on macrobiotic diets. *American Journal of Clinical Nutrition* 50: 818–24.

Dagnelie, Pieter C., Freddy J.V.R.A. Vergote, Wija A. van Staveren, Henk van den Berg, Pieter G. Dingjan, and Joseph G.A.J. Hautvast. 1990. High prevalence of rickets in infants on macrobiotic diets. *American Journal of Clinical Nutrition* 51: 202–208.

Dallman, Peter. R. 1989. Iron deficiency: Does it matter? *Journal of Internal Medicine* 226:5 (November): 367–72.

———. 1993. Nutritional anemias in childhood. In Robert M. Suskind and Leslie Lewinter-Suskind, eds., *Textbook of Pediatric Nutrition,* 2nd ed. New York: Raven Press.

Davis, Adele. 1954. *Let's Eat Right to Keep Fit.* New York: Harcourt, Brace, Jovanovich.

Davis, Julian R., Jr., John Goldenring, and Bertram H. Lubin. 1981. Nutritional vitamin B$_{12}$ deficiency in infants. *American Journal of Diseases of Children* 135: 566–67.

Dawson-Hughes, Bess. 1991. Calcium supplementation and bone loss: A review of controlled clinical trials. *American Journal of Clinical Nutrition* 54 (supplement): 274S–80S.

DeVault, Marjorie L. 1991. *Feeding the Family: The Social Organization of Caring as Gendered Work.* Chicago: University of Chicago Press.

Djoenaidi, W., S. L. H. Notermans, and G. Dunda. 1922. Beriberi cardiomyopathy. *European Journal of Clinical Nutrition* 46: 227–234.

Donovan, Josephine. 1990. Animal rights and feminist theory. *Signs: Journal of Women in Culture and Society* 15: 2 (Winter): 350–75 (reprinted in Gaard 1993).

———. 1992. *Feminist Theory: The Intellectual Traditions of American Feminism.* Expanded edition. New York: Continuum.

———. 1995. Comment on George's "Should Feminists Be Vegetarians?" *Signs: Journal of Women in Culture and Society* 21:1 (Autumn): 226–29.

———. 1996. Attention to suffering: A feminist caring ethic for the treatment of animals. *Journal of Social Philosophy* 27:1 (Spring): 81–102.

Doyle, J. J., A. M. Langevin, and A. Zipursky. 1989. Nutritional vitamin B$_{12}$ deficiency in infancy: Three case reports and a review of the literature. *Pediatric Hematology and Oncology* 6: 161–72.

Dworkin, Andrea. 1974. *Woman Hating.* New York: Dutton/New American Library.

Dworkin, Ronald. 1977. *Taking Rights Seriously.* Cambridge: Harvard University Press.

Dwyer, Johanna T. 1988. Health aspects of vegetarian diets. *American Journal of Clinical Nutrition* 48: 712–38.

———. 1991. Nutritional consequences of vegetarianism. *Annual Reviews in Nutrition* 11: 61–9.

———. 1993a. Nutrition and the adolescent. In Robert M. Suskind and Leslie Lewinter-Suskind, *Textbook of Pediatric Nutrition,* 2nd ed., 257–64. New York: Raven Press.

———. 1993b. Vegetarianism in children. In Patricia M. Queen and Carol E. Lang, eds., *Handbook of Pediatric Nutrition,* 171–86. Gaithersburg, Md.: Aspen Publishers.

———., and Franklin M. Loew. 1994. Nutritional risks of vegan diets to women and children: Are they preventable? *Journal of Agricultural and Environmental Ethics* 7:1 87–109.

———., Linda G. Miller, Nancy L. Arduino, Elizabeth M. Andrew, William H. Dietz, Jr., James C. Reed, and Homer B.C. Reed, Jr. 1980. Mental age and I.Q. of predominantly vegetarian children. *Journal of the American Dietetic Association* 76 (February): 142–47.

———., Ruth Palombo, Halorie Thorne, Isabelle Valadian, and Robert B. Reed. 1978. Preschoolers on alternate life-style diets. *Journal of the American Dietetic Association* 72: 264–70.

Elston, Mary Ann. 1987. Women and anti-vivisection in Victorian England, 1870–1900. In Nicolaas A. Rupke, ed., *Vivisection in Historical Perspective,* 259–294. London and New York: Routledge.

Fairbanks, Virgil F., J. L. Fahey, and B. Ernest. 1971. *Clinical Disorders of Iron Metabolism.* 2nd ed. New York: Gruen & Stratton.

Falciglia, Grace A., and Philippa A. Norton. 1994. Evidence for a genetic influence on preference for some foods. *Journal of the American Dietetic Association* 94(2): 130, 154–58.

Feinberg, Joel. 1973. Human rights. Chapter 6 of *Social Philosophy*, 84–97. Englewood Cliffs, N.J.: Prentice-Hall.

———. 1984. *Harm to Others.* New York: Oxford University Press.

Festa, Melody D., Helen L. Anderson, Richard P. Dowdy, and Mark R. Ellersieck. 1985. Effect of zinc intake on copper excretion and retention in men. *American Journal of Clinical Nutrition* 41(February): 285-92.

Feuerstein, Trisha Lamb, and Marti Kheel. 1991. *Feminists for Animal Rights Bibliography.* Berkeley, Calif.: Feminists for Animal Rights.

Finch, P. J., L. Ang, K. W. Colston, N. Nisbet, and J. D. Maxwell. 1992. Blunted seasonal variation in serum 25-hydroxy vitamin D and increased risk of osteomalacia in vegetarian London Asians. *European Journal of Clinical Nutrition* 46:7 (July): 509–15.

Food and Drug Administration. 1982. Advice on limiting intake of bonemeal. *FDA Drug Bulletin* 12: 5–6.

Foot, Philippa. 1978. Virtues and vices. In her *Virtues and Vices and Other Essays*, 1–18. Berkeley: University of California Press.

Forman, D., F. Sitas, D. G. Newell, A. R. Stacey, J. Boreham, R. Peto, T. C. Campbell, J. Li, and J. Chen. 1990. Geographic association of *Heliocobacter pylori* antibody prevalence and gastric cancer mortality in rural China. *International Journal of Cancer* 46:4 (October 15): 608–11.

Frader, J., B. Reibman, and D. Turkewitz. 1978. Vitamin B$_{12}$ deficiency in strict vegetarians. *New England Journal of Medicine* 299: 1319.

Fraser, Gary E. 1988. Determinants of ischemic heart disease in Seventh-Day Adventists: A review. *American Journal of Clinical Nutrition* 48: 833–36.

Freeland-Graves, Jeanne. 1988. Mineral adequacy of vegetarian diets. *American Journal of Clinical Nutrition* 48: 859–62.

French, Marilyn. 1986. *Beyond Power: Of Women, Men, and Morality.* New York: Ballantine.

Frey, R. G. 1983. *Rights, Killing, and Suffering.* Oxford and New York: Basil Blackwell.

Friedman, Ruth. 1987. *Animal Experimentation and Animal Rights.* Phoenix, Az.: Oryx Press.

Fuller, Margaret. (1845) 1971. *Woman in the Nineteenth Century.* New York: Norton.

Gaard, Greta, ed. 1993. *Ecofeminism: Women, Animals, Nature.* Philadelphia: Temple University Press.

———, and Lori Gruen. 1995. Comment on George's "Should Feminists Be Vegetarians?" *Signs: Journal of Women in Culture and Society* 21:1 (Autumn): 230–41.

Galler, Roberta. 1984. The myth of the perfect body. In Carole S. Vance, ed., *Pleasure and Danger: Exploring Female Sexuality*, pp. 165–72. Hammersmith, England: Pandora Press.

Garcia, J. L. A. 1990. The primacy of the virtuous. *Philosophia* 20:1/2 (July): 69–91.

Gay, Peter. 1966. *Great Ages of Man: The Age of Enlightenment.* New York: Time-Life.

George, Kathryn Paxton. 1990. So animal a human, . . . Or the moral relevance of being and omnivore. *Journal of Agricultural Ethics* 1:3 (Winter): 175–92.

———. 1992. The use and abuse of scientific studies. *Journal of Agricultural and Environmental Ethics* 5(2): 217–33.

———. 1994a. Discrimination and bias in the vegan ideal. *Journal of Agricultural and Environmental Ethics* 7:1 19–28.

———. 1994b. Should feminists be vegetarians? *Signs: Journal of Women in Culture and Society* 19:2 (Winter): 405–34.

———. 1994c. Use and abuse revisited: Response to Pluhar and Varner. *Journal of Agricultural and Environmental Ethics* 7:1 41–76.

———. 1995. Reply to Adams, Donovan, Gruen and Gaard. *Signs* 21:1 (Autumn): 243–60.

Gier, Nicholas F. 1993. Gandhi, *ahimsa,* and the self. *Gandhi Marg* 15:1(April-June): 24–38.

———. 1994. The virtue of nonviolence: A Buddhist perspective. *Seikyo Times* (February): 28–38.

———. 1995. *Ahimsa,* the self, and Postmodernism: Jain, Vedantist, and Buddhist perspectives. *International Philosophical Quarterly* 35:1 (March): 71–86.

Giere, Ronald N. 1991. *Understanding Scientific Reasoning.* 3rd ed. Fort Worth, Tex.: Holt, Rinehart, and Winston, Inc.

Gilligan, Carol. 1977. In a different voice: Women's conceptions of self and morality. *Harvard Educational Review* 47 (November): 481–517.

———. 1982. *In a Different Voice: Psychological Theory and Women's Development.* Cambridge, Mass.: Harvard University Press.

———. 1995. Hearing the difference: Theorizing connection. *Hypatia* 10:2 (Spring): 120–27.

Gilman, Charlotte Perkins. (1915) 1992. *Herland and Selected Stories.* New York: Signet.

Gleason, Sean J. and Janice C. Swanson. 1988. *An Annotated Bibliography of Selected Materials Concerning the Philosophy of Animal Rights.* Beltsville, Md.: U. S. Department of Agriculture, National Agricultural Library, Animal Welfare Information Center.

Goldin, Barry R., and Sherwood L. Gorbach. 1988. Effect of diet on the plasma levels, metabolism, and excretion of estrogens. *American Journal of Clinical Nutrition* 48: 787–90.

Gould, Stephen Jay. 1981. *The Mismeasure of Man.* New York: W. W. Norton.

Grandin, Temple. 1989a. Calmer—Because they're carried. *Beef* (October).

———. 1989b. Where reform is needed: Bob calf handling and veal calf slaughter. *Large Animal Veterinarian* (January-February): 39–40.

Groller, Ingrid. 1990. Parents poll: Do animals have rights? *Parents* Magazine 65:5 (May): 33.

Gruen, Lori. 1993. Dismantling oppression: An analysis of the connection between women and animals. In Greta Gaard, ed., *Ecofeminism: Women, Animals, Nature,* 60–90. Philadelphia: Temple University Press.

Gruzalski, Bart. 1983. The case against raising and killing animals for food. In Harlan B. Miller, ed., *Ethics and Animals*, 251–65.

Gussow, Joan Dye. 1994. Ecology and vegetarian considerations: Does environmental responsibility demand the elimination of livestock? *American Journal of Clinical Nutrition* 59 (supplement): 1110S–1116S.

Hambidge, K. M., C. Hambidge, M. Jacobs, and J. D. Baum. 1972. Low levels of zinc in hair, anorexia, poor growth, and hypogensia in children. *Pediatric Research* 6: 868–74.

Hamilton, Eva May Nunnelley, Eleanor Noss Whitney, and Frances Sienkiewicz Sizer. 1984. Controversy: World hunger. Chapter 6 in *Nutrition: Concepts and Controversies*. 3rd ed. St. Paul: West Publishing Co.

Harding, Sandra. 1991. *Whose Science? Whose Knowledge?* Ithaca, N.Y.: Cornell University Press.

Hare, R. M. 1981. *Moral Thinking: Its Levels, Method, and Point.* Oxford: Clarendon Press.

Harrison, Ruth. 1964. *Animal Machines: The New Factory Farming Industry.* London: Stuart.

Harsanyi, John C. 1982. Morality and the theory of rational behavior. In Amartya Sen and Bernard Williams, eds., *Utilitarianism and Beyond.* Cambridge: Cambridge University Press.

Hartz, S. C., and J. Blumberg. 1986. Use of vitamin and mineral supplements by the elderly. *Clinical Nutrition* 5: 130–36.

Havala, Suzanne, and Johanna T. Dwyer. 1988. Position of the American Dietetic Association: Vegetarian diets—Technical support paper. *Journal of the American Dietetic Association* 88:3 (March): 352–55.

———. 1993. Position of the American Dietetic Association: Vegetarian diets. *Journal of the American Dietetic Association* 93:11 (November): 1317–19.

Hegsted, D. M. 1986. Calcium and osteoporosis. *Journal of Nutrition* 116: 2316–319.

Held, Virginia. 1984. The obligations of mothers and fathers. In Joyce Trebilcot, ed., *Mothering: Essays in Feminist Theory.* Totowa, N.J.: Rowman & Allanheld.

———. 1987. Feminism and moral theory. In Eva Kittay and Diana Meyers, eds., *Women and Moral Theory.* Savage, Md.: Rowman & Littlefield.

———. 1990. Feminist transformations of moral theory. *Philosophy and Phenomenological Research* 50 (supplement): 321–44.

———. 1993. *Feminist Morality: Transforming Culture, Society, and Politics.* Chicago: University of Chicago Press.

———. 1995. The meshing of care and justice. *Hypatia* 10:2 (Spring): 128–32.

Heldke, Lisa M. 1988. Recipes for theory making. *Hypatia* 3:2 (reprinted in Curtin and Heldke 1992).

———. 1992a. Food politics, political food. In Deane W. Curtin and Lisa M. Heldke, eds., *Cooking, Eating, Thinking: Transformative Philosophies of Food.* Bloomington: Indiana University Press.

———. 1992b. Foodmaking as a thoughtful practice. In Deane W. Curtin and Lisa M. Heldke, eds., *Cooking, Eating, Thinking: Transformative Philosophies of Food.* Bloomington: Indiana University Press.

Henderson, J. B., M. G. Dunnigan, W. B. McIntosh, A. A. Abdul-Motaal, and D. Hole. 1990. Asian osteomalacia is determined by dietary factors when exposure to ultraviolet radiation is restricted: A risk factor model. *Quarterly Journal of Medicine* 75: 923–33.

Henderson, J. B., M. G. Dunnigan, W. B. McIntosh, A. A. Abdul-Motaal, G. Gettingby, and B. M. Glekin. 1987. The importance of limited exposure to ultraviolet radiation and dietary factors in the aetiology of Asian rickets: A risk factor model. *Quarterly Journal of Medicine* 63: 405–12.

Herbert, Victor. 1980. Laetrile: Cult of cyanide. In *Nutrition Cultism*, 15–74. Philadelphia, Penn.: George F. Stickley.

———. 1984. Vitamin B_{12}. In *Nutrition Reviews' Present Knowledge in Nutrition*. 5th ed., 347–64. Washington, D.C.: The Nutrition Foundation.

———. 1988. Vitamin B_{12}: Plant sources, requirements, assay. *American Journal of Clinical Nutrition* 48: 852–58.

———, and Genell J. Subak-Sharpe, eds. 1990. *The Mount Sinai School of Medicine Complete Book of Nutrition*. New York: St. Martin's Press.

Hercberg, Serge, and Pilar Galan. 1989. Biochemical effects of iron deprivation. *Acta Paediatrica Scandinavica* 361 (supplement): 63–70.

———. 1992. Nutritional anaemias. *Baillière's Clinical Haematology* 5:1 (January): 143–68.

Hernandez-Avila, Mauricio, Graham A. Colditz, Meir J. Stampfer, Bernard Rosner, Frank E. Speizer, and Walter C. Willett. 1991. Caffeine, moderate alcohol intake, and risk of fractures of the hip and forearm in middle-aged women. *American Journal of Clinical Nutrition* 54: 157–63.

Heyes, Cressida J. 1997. Anti-essentialism in practice: Carol Gilligan and feminist philosophy. *Hypatia* 12:3 (Summer): 142–63.

Higginbottom, M.C., L. Sweetman, and W. L. Nyhan. 1978. A syndrome of methylmalonic aciduria, homocystinuria, megaloblastic anemia and neurologic abnormalities in a vitamin B_{12}-deficient breast-fed infant of a strict vegetarian. *New England Journal of Medicine* 299: 317–23.

Hino, S. 1989. Milk-borne transmission of HTLV-1 as a major route in the endemic cycle. *Acta Paediatrica Japonica* 31: 428–35.

Hittinger, Russell. 1989. After MacIntyre: Natural law theory, virtue ethics, and *eudaimonia*. *International Philosophical Quarterly* 29:4 (December): 449–461.

Hoagland, Sarah Lucia. 1990. Some concerns about Nel Noddings' *Caring*. *Hypatia* 5:1 (Spring): 109–14.

Hoey, H., J. C. Linnell, V. G. Oberholzer, and B. M. Laurence. 1982. Vitamin B_{12} deficiency in a breastfed infant of a mother with pernicious anemia. *Journal of the Royal Society of Medicine* (London) 75: 656–58.

Holick, Michael F., Qing Shao, Wen Wei Liu, and Tai C. Chen. 1992. The vitamin D content of fortified milk and infant formula. *The New England Journal of Medicine* 326 (April 30): 1178–81.

Holloway, Marguerite, and Philip Yam. 1992. Reflecting differences: Health care begins to address the needs of women and minorities. *Scientific American* (March): 13–18.

Houston, Barbara. 1990. Caring and exploitation. *Hypatia* 5:1 (Spring): 115–19.

Hu, Ji-Fan, Xi-He Zhao, Jian-Bin Jia, Banoo Parpia, and T. Colin Campbell. 1993. Dietary calcium and bone density among middle-aged and elderly women in China. *American Journal of Clinical Nutrition* 58: 219–27.

Institute of Medicine. 1990. *Nutrition during Pregnancy.* Subcommittee on Nutritional Status and Weight Gain during Pregnancy, Subcommittee on Dietary Intakes and Nutrient Supplements during Pregnancy, Committee on Nutritional Status during Pregnancy and Lactation, Food and Nutrition Board, National Academy of Sciences. Washington, D.C.: National Academy Press.

———. 1991. *Nutrition during Lactation.* Subcommittee on Nutrition during Lactation, Committee on Nutritional Status during Pregnancy and Lactation, Food and Nutrition Board, National Academy of Sciences. Washington, D.C.: National Academy Press.

Jacobs, Cathy, and Johanna T. Dwyer. 1988. Vegetarian children: Appropriate and inappropriate diets. *American Journal of Clinical Nutrition* 48: 811–18.

Jaggar, Alison M. 1990. Sexual difference and sexual equality. In Deborah L. Rhode, ed., *Theoretical Perspectives on Sexual Difference*, 239–54, 302–03. New Haven: Yale University Press.

———. 1991. Feminist ethics: Projects, problems, prospects. In Claudia Card, ed., *Feminist Ethics.* Lawrence: University of Kansas Press.

Johns Hopkins Medical Institutions. 1994a. Our readers ask: Does lifting weights help fight the bone loss of osteoporosis? *The Johns Hopkins Medical Letter: Health after 50* 5:11 (January): 8.

Johns Hopkins Medical Institutions. 1994b. Calcium: Maximizing its benefit. *The Johns Hopkins Medical Letter: Health after 50* 5:12 (February): 4–5.

Johns Hopkins Medical Institutions. 1994c. Osteoporosis: No sex discrimination. *Johns Hopkins Medical Letter: Health after 50* 6:1 (March): 3.

Johnson, P. R., and J. S. Roloff. 1982. Vitamin B_{12} deficiency in an infant strictly breast-fed by a mother with latent pernicious anemia. *Journal of Pediatrics* 100: 917–19.

Johnston, Patricia K. 1994. Preface [to Second International Congress on Vegetarian Nutrition]. *American Journal of Clinical Nutrition* 59 (supplement): vii.

Jones, W. T. 1969. *A History of Western Philosophy*, vol. 2: *The Medieval Mind.* 2nd ed. New York: Harcourt, Brace, Jovanovich.

Journal of the American Medical Association. 1974. Medical news: Babies who eat no animal protein fail to grow at normal rate. *Journal of the American Medical Association* 228:6 (May 6): 675–76.

Kahane, Howard. 1984. *Logic and Contemporary Rhetoric: The Use of Reason in Everyday Life.* 4th ed. Belmont, Calif.: Wadsworth.

Kalucy, Ross S. 1987. The "new" nutrition. *Medical Journal of Australia* 147: 529–30.

Kanis, J. A. 1993. The incidence of hip fracture in Europe. *Osteoporosis International (England)* 3 (supplement): 10–15.

Kant, Immanuel. (1780) 1963. *Lectures on Ethics.* Trans. Louis Infield. New York: Harper and Row.

———. (1785) 1969. *Foundations of the Metaphysics of Morals.* Text and critical essays edited by Robert Paul Wolff. Trans. Lewis White Beck. Indianapolis: Bobbs-Merrill.

————. (1788) 1956. *Critique of Practical Reason*. Trans. Lewis White Beck. Indianapolis: Bobbs-Merrill.

Kantha, Sachi Sri. 1990. Nutrition and health in China, 1949 to 1989. *Progress in Food and Nutrition Science* 14: 93–137.

Karjalainen, Jukka, Julio M. Martin, Mikael Knip, Jorma Ilonen, Brian H. Robinson, Erkki Savilahti, Hans K. Akerblom, and Hans-Michael Dosch. 1992. A bovine albumin peptide as a possible trigger of insulin-dependent diabetes mellitus. *The New England Journal of Medicine* 327:5 (July 30): 302–307.

Kay, Herma Hill. 1985. Equality and difference: The case of pregnancy. *Berkeley Women's Law Journal* 1: 1–37 (reprinted in Smith 1993).

Kaye, Howard L. 1986. *The Social Meaning of Modern Biology: From Social Darwinism to Sociobiology*. New Haven and London: Yale University Press.

Keller, Evelyn Fox. 1982. Feminism and science. *Signs* 7:3 (Spring): 589–602.

Keller, Jean. 1997. Autonomy, relationality, and feminist ethics. *Hypatia* 12:2 (Spring): 152–64.

Kheel, Marti. 1985. The liberation of nature: A circular affair. *Environmental Ethics* 7 (Summer): 135–49.

Klingshirn, L. A., R. R. Pate, S. P. Bourque, J. M. Davis, and R. G. Sargent. 1992. Effect of iron supplementation on endurance capacity in iron-depleted female runners. *Medicine and Science in Sports and Exercise* 24:7 (July): 819–24.

Kohlberg, Lawrence. 1969. Stage and sequence: The cognitive-development approach to socialization. In D. A. Goslin, ed., *Handbook of Socialization Theory and Research*. Chicago: Rand McNally.

————. 1971. From is to ought: How to commit the naturalistic fallacy and get away with it in the study of moral development. In T. Mischel, ed., *Cognitive Development and Epistemology*. New York: Academic Press.

————, and R. Kramer. 1969. Continuities and discontinuities in child and adult moral development. *Human Development* 12: 93–120.

Kozol, Jonathan. 1988. *Rachel and Her Children: Homeless Families in America*. New York: Crown.

Kroeger-Mappes, Joy. 1994. The ethic of care vis-à-vis the ethic of rights: A problem for contemporary moral theory. *Hypatia* 9:3 (Summer): 108–31.

Kuhne T., R. Bubl, and R. Baumgartner. 1991. Maternal vegan diet causing a serious infantile neurological disorder due to vitamin B_{12} deficiency. *European Journal of Pediatrics* 150: 205–08.

Kuhse, Helga, Peter Singer, and Maurice Rickard. 1998. Reconciling impartial morality and a feminist ethic of care. *Journal of Value Inquiry* 32: 451–63.

Kultgen, John. 1998a. The vicissitudes of common-sense virtue ethics, Part I: From Aristotle to Slote. *Journal of Value Inquiry* 32: 325–41.

————. 1998b. The vicissitudes of common-sense virtue ethics, Part II: The heuristic use of common sense. *Journal of Value Inquiry* 32: 465–78.

Lacroix, J., M. A. Machter, J. Badoual, and G. Huault. 1981. Complications of a vegetarian diet in a breast-fed girl. *Archives Françaises de Pediatrie (Paris)* 38: 233–38.

Lampkin, B.C., and E. F. Saunders. 1969. Nutritional vitamin B_{12} deficiency in an infant. *Journal of Pediatrics* 75: 1053–55.

————, N. A. Shore, and D. Chadwick. 1966. Megaloblastic anemia of infancy secondary to pernicious anemia. *New England Journal of Medicine* 274: 1168–71.

Lappé, Frances Moore. 1971. *Diet for a Small Planet.* New York: Ballantine.

————. 1982. *Diet for a Small Planet.* 10th ed. New York: Ballantine.

————, and Joseph Collins. 1986. *World Hunger: Twelve Myths.* New York: Grove Press.

Latham, M. C., L. S. Stephenson, S. N. Kinoti, M. S. Zaman, and K. M. Kurz. 1990. Improvements in growth following iron supplementation in young Kenyan school children. *Nutrition* 6:2 (March-April): 159–65.

Lebrun, John B., Michael E. K. Moffatt, Ronald J. T. Mundy, Robert K. Sangster, Brian D. Postl, Joseph P. Dooley, Louise A. Dilling, John C. Godel, and James C. Haworth. 1993. Vitamin D deficiency in a Manitoba community. *Canadian Journal of Public Health* 84: 394–96.

Lewis, Stephen. 1994. An opinion on the global impact of meat consumption. *American Journal of Clinical Nutrition* 59 (supplement): 1099S–1102S.

Liebman, Bonnie. 1992. Crying over milk. *Nutrition Action Health Letter* 19:10 (December): 1-2.

————. 1993. Calcium: Not unleaded. *Nutrition Action Health Letter* 20:10 (December): 4.

————. 1994. Non-trivial pursuits: Playing the research game. *Nutrition Action Health Letter* 21:8 (October): 1, 7–9.

Linzey, Andrew. 1987. *Christianity and the Rights of Animals.* New York: Crossroad.

Littleton, Christine A. 1987. Reconstructing sexual equality. *California Law Review* 75 (4): 1279–1337.

Lloyd, Genevieve. 1984. *The Man of Reason: "Male" and "Female" in Western Philosophy.* Minneapolis: University of Minnesota Press.

Logue, Alexandra W. 1986. *The Psychology of Eating and Drinking.* New York: W. H. Freeman.

Löwik, Michiel R. H., Karin F. A. M. Hulshof, Petra Schneijder, Jaap Schrijver, Ann A. M. Colen, and Paul van Houten. 1993. Vitamin C status in elderly women: A comparison between women living in a nursing home and women living independently. *Journal of the American Dietetic Association* 93:2 (February): 167–72.

Löwik, M. R., J. Schrijver, J. Odink, H. van den Berg, and M. Wedel. 1990. Long-term effects of a vegetarian diet on the nutritional status of elderly people. *Journal of the American College of Nutrition* 9: 600–09.

Lutz, J., and R. Tesar. 1990. Mother-daughter pairs: Spinal and femoral bone density and dietary intakes. *American Journal of Clinical Nutrition* 52: 872–77.

McCloskey, H. J. 1979. Moral rights and animals. *Inquiry* 22(1): 23–54 (reprinted in Richard A. Wasserstrom, ed., *Today's Moral Problems,* 3rd ed. New York: Macmillan).

McDonald, Janet T. 1986. Vitamin and mineral supplement use in the United States. *Clinical Nutrition* 5: 27–33.

McDonald, R., and C. L. Keen. 1988. Iron, zinc and magnesium nutrition and athletic performance. *Sports Medicine* 5:3 (May): 171–84.

MacIntyre, Alasdair. 1981. *After Virtue.* Notre Dame, Ind.: University of Notre Dame Press.

————. 1984. *After Virtue.* 2nd ed. Notre Dame, Ind.: University of Notre Dame Press.

————. 1988. *Sóphrosuné:* How a virtue can become socially disruptive. *Midwest Studies in Philosophy,* vol. 13: Ethical Theory: *Character and Virtue.* Notre Dame, Ind.: University of Notre Dame Press.

MacKinnon, Catherine. 1985. Pornography, civil rights, and speech. *Harvard Civil Rights-Civil Liberties Law Review* 20:1 (Winter): 1–70.

————. 1979. *Sexual Harassment of Working Women: A Case of Sex Discrimination.* New Haven: Yale University Press.

————. 1989. *Toward a Feminist Theory of the State.* Cambridge: Harvard University Press (portions reprinted in Smith 1993).

McMurray, Richard J. 1991. Gender disparities in clinical decision-making. *Code of Medical Ethics Reports.* Council on Ethical and Judicial Affairs, American Medical Association.

MacSween, Morag. 1993. *Anorexic Bodies: A Feminist and Sociological Perspective on Anorexia Nervosa.* New York: Routledge.

Magel, Charles R. 1981. *A Bibliography on Animal Rights and Related Matters.* Washington, D.C.: University Press of America.

————. 1989. *Keyguide to Information Sources in Animal Rights.* Jefferson, N.C.: McFarland.

Mangels, Ann Reed, and Suzanne Havala. 1994. Vegan diets for women, infants, and children. *Journal of Agricultural and Environmental Ethics* 7(1): 111–22.

Mason, Jim, and Peter Singer. 1980. *Animal Factories.* New York: Crown.

Matkovic, Velimir K., K. Kostial, I. Simonovic, R. Buzina, A. Broderac, and B. E. C. Nordin. 1979. Bone status and fracture rates in two regions of Yugoslavia. *American Journal of Clinical Nutrition* 32: 540–49.

Melby, C. L., D. G. Goldflies, and M. L. Toohey. 1993. Blood pressure differences in older Black and white long-term vegetarians and nonvegetarians. *Journal of the American College of Nutrition* 12:3 (June): 262–69.

Meyer, Michael. 1992. National affairs: Los Angeles will save itself. *Newsweek* 119:20 (May 18): 46.

Meyers, Diana Tietjens. 1989. *Self, Society, and Personal Choice.* New York: Columbia University Press.

————. 1993. Moral reflection: Beyond impartial reason. *Hypatia* 8:3 (Summer): 21–47.

Michaud, J. L., B. Lemieux, H. Ogier, and M. A. Lambert. 1992. Nutritional vitamin B_{12} deficiency: Two cases detected by routine newborn urinary screening. *European Journal of Pediatrics* 151:3 (March): 218–20.

Midgley, Mary. 1983a. *Animals and Why They Matter.* Athens: University of Georgia Press.

————. 1983b. Duties concerning islands. *Encounter* 60 (February): 36–43.

Mill, John Stuart. (1859) 1974. *On Liberty.* In Mary Warnock, ed., *John Stuart Mill: Utilitarianism, On Liberty, Essay on Bentham.* New York: New American Library.

————. (1863) 1974. *Utilitarianism.* In Mary Warnock, ed., *John Stuart Mill: Utilitarianism, On Liberty, Essay on Bentham.* New York: New American Library.

————. 1869. *The Subjection of Women.* London: Longmans, Green, Reader, & Dyer.

Mirrlees, J. A. 1982. The economic uses of utilitarianism. In Amartya Sen and Bernard Williams, eds., *Utilitarianism and Beyond.* Cambridge: Cambridge University Press.

Monfort-Gouraud, M., A Bongiorno, M. A. Le Gall, and J. Badoual. 1993. Severe megaloblastic anemia in child breast fed by a vegetarian mother. *Annales de Pediatrie (Paris)* 40(1): 28–31.

Monro, D. H. 1967. Jeremy Bentham. In Paul Edwards, ed., *The Encyclopedia of Philosophy,* vol. 1, 280–285. New York: Macmillan.

Montague, Phillip. 1992. Virtue ethics: A qualified success story. *American Philosophical Quarterly* 29:1 (January): 53–61.

Morgan, Kathryn Pauly. 1991. Women and the knife: Cosmetic surgery and the colonization of women's bodies. *Hypatia* 6:3 (Fall): 25–53.

Morgan, Robin. 1982. Metaphysical feminism. In Charlene Spretnak, ed., *The Politics of Women's Spirituality.* Garden City, N.Y.: Anchor Press.

Morrison, N. A., C. J. Qi, and A. Tokita. 1994. Prediction of bone density from vitamin D receptor alleles. *Nature* 367 (January 20): 284–87.

Moss, A. J., A. S. Levy, I. Kim, and Y. K. Park. 1989. Use of vitamin and mineral supplements in the United States: Current users, types of products, and nutrients. *Advance Data in Vital Health Statistics* 174. (National Center for Health Statistics)

Mundy, Gregory R. 1994. Boning up on genes. *Nature* 367 (January 20): 216–17.

Munro, Hamish N., Paulo M. Suter, and Robert M. Russell. 1987. Nutritional requirements of the elderly. *Annual Review of Nutrition* 7: 23–49.

Mutch, Patricia B. 1988. Food guides for the vegetarian. *American Journal of Clinical Nutrition* 48:3 (September): 913–19.

National Nutrition Consortium, Inc. 1978. *Vitamin-Mineral Safety, Toxicity and Misuse.* Chicago: The American Dietetic Association.

National Research Council. 1989a. *Diet and Health: Implications for Reducing Chronic Disease Risk.* Committee on Diet and Health, Food and Nutrition Board, Commission on Life Sciences. Washington, D.C.: National Academy Press.

————. 1989b. *Recommended Dietary Allowances.* 10th ed. Subcommittee on the Tenth Edition of the RDAs, Food and Nutrition Board, Commission on Life Sciences. Washington, D.C.: National Academy Press.

Nicoll, Charles S., and Sharon M. Russell. 1991. Mozart, Alexander the Great, and the animal rights/liberation philosophy. *FASEB Journal* 5 (November): 2888–92.

Nieman, David C. 1988. Vegetarian dietary practices and endurance performance. *American Journal of Clinical Nutrition* 48: 754–61.

Noddings, Nel. 1984. *Caring: A Feminine Approach to Ethics and Moral Education.* Berkeley: University of California Press.

————. 1990. A response. *Hypatia* 5:1 (Spring): 120–26.

Nordin, B. E. C. 1966. International patterns of osteoporosis. *Clinical Orthopedics* 45: 17–30.

Nordquist, Joan. 1991. *Animal Rights: A Bibliography*. Santa Cruz, Calif.: Reference and Research Services.

Norgaard, Richard B. 1987. The epistemological basis of agroecology. In Miguel A. Altieri, ed., *Agroecology: The Scientific Basis of Alternative Agriculture*. Boulder: Westview.

Nozick, Robert. 1974. *Anarchy, State, Utopia*. Basic Books, Inc.

O'Connell, Joan M., Michael J. Dibley, Janet Sierra, Barbara Wallace, James S. Marks, and Ray Yip. 1989. Growth of vegetarian children: The Farm study. *Pediatrics* 84:3 (September): 475–81.

O'Connor, Maureen A., Steven W. Touyz, Stewart M. Dunn, and Pierre J. V. Beaumont. 1987. Vegetarianism in anorexia nervosa? A review of 116 consecutive cases. *The Medical Journal of Australia* 147: 540–42.

Olejer, Victoria L. 1993. Food hypersensitivities. In Patricia M. Queen and Carol E. Lang, eds., *Handbook of Pediatric Nutrition*. Gaithersburg, Md.: Aspen.

Ornish, Dean. 1993. Can lifestyle changes reverse coronary heart disease? *World Review of Nutrition and Dietetics* 72: 38–48.

Oski, Frank A. 1993. Current concepts: Iron deficiency in infancy and childhood. *New England Journal of Medicine* 329(3): 190–93.

Ossell, Joanne, [M.S., R.D.]. 1993. *Food Analyst Plus: A Complete Nutritional Analysis Software*. CD-ROM. Hopkins, Minn.: Hopkins Technology.

Palacio, Joseph. 1991. Kin ties, food, and remittances in a Garifuna village in southern Belize. In Anne Sharman, Janet Theophano, Karen Curtis, and Ellen Messer, eds., *Diet and Domestic Life in Society*, 119–146. Philadelphia: Temple University Press.

Parks, Y. A., and B. A. Wharton. 1989. Iron deficiency and the brain. *Acta Paediatrica Scandinavica* 361 (supplement): 71–77.

Patlak, Margie. 1993. Probing the link between ethnic origin and disease. *National Research Council NewsReport* 43:2 (Spring): 18–20.

Peacock, Munro. 1991. Calcium absorption efficiency and calcium requirements in children and adolescents. *American Journal of Clinical Nutrition* 54 (supplement): 261S–265S.

Peikin, Steven. 1991. *Gastrointestinal Health*. New York: Harper Perennial.

Perkin, Judy, and Stephanie F. McCann. 1984. Food for ethnic Americans: Is the government trying to turn the melting pot into a one-dish dinner? In Linda Keller Brown and Kay Mussel, eds., *Ethnic and Regional Foodways in the United States: The Performance of Group Identity*, 238–58. Knoxville: University of Tennessee Press.

Pertschuk, Michael J. 1993. Nutritional considerations in the treatment of anorexia nervosa and bulima. In Robert M. Suskind and Leslie Lewinter-Suskind, *Textbook of Pediatric Nutrition*, 2nd ed. New York: Raven Press.

Phillips, Spencer, N. Fox, J. Jacobs, and W. E. Wright. 1988. The direct medical costs of osteoporosis for American women aged 45 and older, 1986. *Bone* 9: 271–79.

Physicians Committee for Responsible Medicine (PCRM). 1991. The new four food groups. *PCRM Update* (May-June): 1–11.

Pincoffs, Edmund L. 1986. *Quandries and Virtues: Against Reductivism in Ethics*. Lawrence: University Press of Kansas.

Plato. 1961. *The Collected Dialogues.* Edited by Edith Hamilton and Huntington Cairns, trans. Lane Cooper. Princeton, N.J.: Princeton University Press.

Pluhar, Evelyn. 1988a. Is there a morally relevant difference between human and animal nonpersons? *Journal of Agricultural Ethics* 1: 59–68.

———. 1988b. When is it morally acceptable to kill animals? *Journal of Agricultural Ethics* 1: 211–224.

———. 1992. Who can be morally obligated to be a vegetarian? *Journal of Agricultural and Environmental Ethics* 5(2): 189–215.

———. 1993. On vegetarianism, morality, and science: A counter-reply. *Journal of Agricultural and Environmental Ethics* 6:2 (Summer): 21–49.

———. 1994. Vegetarianism, morality, and science revisited. *Journal of Agricultural and Environmental Ethics* 7(1): 77–82.

Plumwood, Val. 1991. Nature, self, and gender: Feminism, environmental philosophy, and the critique of rationalism. *Hypatia* 6:1 (Spring): 3–27.

Pocock, N.A., J. A. Eisman, J. L. Hopper, M. G. Yeates, P. N. Sambrook, and S. Ebert. 1987. Genetic determinants of bone mass in adults: A twin study. *Journal of Clinical Investigation* 80: 706–10.

Pollitzer, William S., and John J. B. Anderson. 1989. Ethnic and genetic differences in bone mass: A review with a hereditary versus environmental perspective. *American Journal of Clinical Nutrition* 50: 1244–59.

Prasad, A. S. 1982. Clinical and biochemical spectrum of zinc deficiency in human subjects. In A. S. Prasad, ed. *Clinical, Biochemical, and Nutritional Aspects of Trace Elements*, vol. 6., *Current Topics in Nutrition and Disease*, 3–62. New York: Alan R. Liss.

Probart, C. K., and L. S. Lieberman. 1992. Body image disturbances in women. *Collegium Antropologicum* 16(1): 151–56.

Queen, Patricia M., and Carol E. Lang, eds. 1993. *Handbook of Pediatric Nutrition.* Gaithersburg, Md.: Aspen.

Rachels, James. 1986. *The Elements of Moral Philosophy.* New York: Random House.

———. 1990. *Created from Animals: The Moral Implications of Darwinism.* New York: Oxford University Press.

Rawls, John. 1971. *A Theory of Justice.* Cambridge, Mass.: Harvard University Press.

Regan, Tom. 1983. *The Case for Animal Rights.* Berkeley: University of California Press.

———, ed. 1986. *Animal Sacrifices: Religious Perspectives on the Use of Animals in Science*, 3–14. Philadelphia: Temple University Press.

———. 1991. *The Thee Generation: Reflections on the Coming Revolution.* Philadelphia: Temple University Press.

Rendle-Short, J., J. R. Tiernan, and S. Hagwood. 1979. Vegan mothers with vitamin B_{12} deficiency. *Medical Journal of Australia* 2: 483.

Rizvi, Najma. 1991. Socioeconomic and cultural factors affecting interhousehold and intrahousehold food distribution in rural and urban Bangladesh. In Anne Sharman, Janet Theophano, Karen Curtis, and Ellen Messer, eds., *Diet and Domestic Life in Society*, 91–118. Philadelphia: Temple University Press.

Robbins, John. 1987. *Diet for a New America.* Walpole, N.H.: Stillpoint.

Robertson, Laurel, Carol Flinders, and Brian Ruppenthal. 1986. *The New Laurel's Kitchen.* Berkeley: Ten Speed Press.

Rodysill, Kirk J. 1987. Postmenopausal osteoporosis—Intervention and prophylaxis. A review. *Journal of Chronic Diseases* 40(8) :743–60.

Rollin, Bernard E. 1981. *Animal Rights and Human Morality.* Buffalo: Prometheus.

———. 1989. *The Unheeded Cry: Animal Consciousness, Animal Pain and Science.* New York: Oxford University Press.

Rose, David P., Madeleine Goldman, Jeanne M. Connolly, and Leslie E. Strong. 1991. High-fiber diet reduces serum estrogen concentrations in premenopausal women. *American Journal of Clinical Nutrition* 54: 520–25.

Rowland, T. W. 1990. Iron deficiency in the young athlete. *Pediatric Clinics of North America* 37:5 (October): 1153–63.

Royall, Richard M. 1991. Ethics and statistics in randomized clinical trials. *Statistical Science* 6(1): 52–88.

Ruddick, Sara. 1989. *Maternal Thinking: Toward a Politics of Peace.* Boston: Beacon.

Ruether, Rosemary Radford. 1975. *New Woman/New Earth: Sexist Ideologies and Human Liberation.* New York: Seabury.

Sadowitz, P.D., A. Livingston, and R. M. Cavanaugh. 1986. Developmental regression as an early manifestation of vitamin B_{12} deficiency. *Clinical Pediatrics* 25: 369–71.

Salomone, Constantia. 1982. The prevalence of the natural law: Women and animal rights. In Pam McAllister, ed., *Reweaving the Web of Life: Feminism and Nonviolence,* pp. 364–75. Philadelphia: New Society.

Salonen, J. T., K. Nyyssönen, H. Korpela, J. Tuomilehto, R. Seppänen, and R. Salonen. 1992. High stored-iron levels are associated with excess risk of myocardial infarction in eastern Finnish men. *Circulation* 86: 803–81.

Salt, Henry S. (1892) 1980. *Animals' Rights Considered in Relation to Social Progress.* Clarks Summit, Pa.: Society for Animal Rights, Inc.

Saltman, Paul, Joel Gurin, and Ira Mothner. 1987. *The California Nutrition Book.* Boston: Little, Brown.

Sanders, T.A.B., and Sheela Reddy. 1994. Vegetarian diets and children. *American Journal of Clinical Nutrition* 59 (supplement): S1176–S1181.

Sandler, Rivka Black, Charles W. Slemenda, Ronald E. LaPorte, Jane A. Cauley, Margaret M. Schramm, Mary Lynn Barresi, and Andrea M. Kriska. 1985. Postmenopausal bone density and milk consumption in childhood and adolescence. *American Journal of Clinical Nutrition* 42 (August): 270–74.

Sapontzis, Steve F. 1987. *Morals, Reasons, and Animals.* Philadelphia: Temple University Press.

Savage-Rumbaugh, E. S., and D. M. Rumbaugh. 1978a. Symbolic communication between two chimpanzees. *Science* 201: 641–44.

———. 1978b. Symbolization, language, and chimpanzees: a theoretical re-evaluation based on mutual language acquisition processes in four young *Pan troglodytes. Brain and Language* 6: 265–300.

Savage-Rumbaugh, E. S., D. M. Rumbaugh, and S. Boyson. 1978. Linguistically mediated tool use and exchange by chimpanzees (*Pan troglodytes*). *Behavioral and Brain Sciences* 1: 539–54.

Scales, Ann C. 1986. The emergence of feminist jurisprudence: An essay. *Yale Law Journal* 95: 1373–1403 (reprinted in Smith 1993).

Schardt, David. 1993. The problem with protein. *Nutrition Action Health Letter* 20:5 (June): 5–7.

Scheffler, Samuel, ed. 1988. *Consequentialism and Its Critics*. Oxford: Oxford University Press.

Schneewind, J. B. 1990. The misfortunes of virtue. *Ethics* 101 (October): 42–63.

Schnitzler, Christine M., John M. Pettifor, Deepak Patel, Julia M. Mesquita, Gopal P. Moodley, and Dianne Zachen. 1994. Metabolic bone disease in Black teenagers with genu valgum or varum without radiologic rickets: A bone histomorphometric study. *Journal of Bone and Mineral Research* 9(4): 479–86.

Scrimshaw, Nevin S. 1991. Iron deficiency. *Scientific American* (October): 46–52.

———. 1990. Nutrition: Prospects for the 1990s. *Annual Review of Public Health* 11: 53–68.

Seligmann, Jean with Lynda Wright. 1988. How to handle an elephant: Zoos and animal abuse. *Newsweek* (November 14): 71.

Sen, Amartya, and Bernard Williams. 1982. Introduction: Utilitarianism and beyond. In Amartya Sen and Bernard Williams, eds., *Utilitarianism and Beyond*. Cambridge: Cambridge University Press.

Sharma, D. C., V. Pendse, K. Sahay, and B. L. Soni. 1991. The changing pattern of maternal and neonatal anaemia at Udaipur during two decades in relation to poverty, parity, prematurity, and vegetarianism. *Asia Oceania Journal of Obstetrics and Gynecology* 17:1 (March): 13–17.

Sharma, Vinit, and Anuragini Sharma. 1992. Health profile of pregnant adolescents among selected tribal populations in Rajasthan, India. 1992. *Journal of Adolescent Health* 13: 696–699.

Sharman, Anne. 1991. From generation to generation: Resources, experience, and orientation in the dietary patterns of selected urban American households. In Anne Sharman, Janet Theophano, Karen Curtis, and Ellen Messer, eds., *Diet and Domestic Life in Society*, 173–204. Philadelphia: Temple University Press.

———, Janet Theophano, Karen Curtis, and Ellen Messer, eds. 1991. *Diet and Domestic Life in Society*. Philadelphia: Temple University Press.

Sherwin, Susan. 1989. Feminist and medical ethics: Two different approaches to contextual ethics. *Hypatia* 4:2 (Summer).

Shiva, Vandana. 1989. *Staying Alive: Women, Ecology, and Development*. London: Zed Books.

———. 1991. *The Violence of the Green Revolution: Third World Agriculture, Ecology, and Politics*. London: Zed Books.

Shull, Margaret W., Robert B. Reed, Isabelle Valadian, Ruth Palombo, Halorie Thorne, and Johanna T. Dwyer. 1977. Velocities of growth in vegetarian pre-school children. *Pediatrics* 60:4 (October): 410–17.

Silberstein, E. P., R. G. Wilson, and J. M. Surlock. 1987. Methylmalonic aciduria in an infant of a mother with undiagnosed pernicious anemia. *Medical Journal of Australia* 146: 329–330.

Simoons, F. J. 1982. A geographic approach to senile cataracts. *Digestive Diseases and Sciences* 27(3): 257–64.

Singer, Peter. 1975. *Animal Liberation.* New York: Avon.

———. 1979. Killing humans and killing animals. *Inquiry* 22: 145–56.

———. 1981. *The Expanding Circle: Ethics and Sociobiology.* New York: Farrar, Straus & Giroux.

———. 1986. Animals and the value of life. In Tom Regan, ed., *Matters of Life and Death: New Introductory Essays in Moral Philosophy,* 2nd ed. New York: Random House.

———. 1990. *Animal Liberation.* 2nd ed. New York: Random House.

Sklar, R. 1986. Nutritional vitamin B_{12} deficiency in a breast-fed infant of a vegan-diet mother. *Clinical Pediatrics* 25: 219–21.

Slote, Michael. 1985. *Common-Sense Morality and Consequentialism.* London: Routledge & Kegan Paul.

———. 1992. *From Morality to Virtue.* Oxford: Oxford University Press.

Smart, J. J. C., and Bernard Williams. 1973. *Utilitarianism: For and Against.* Cambridge: Cambridge University Press.

Smith, Patricia, ed. 1993. *Feminist Jurisprudence.* New York: Oxford University Press.

Smith, Roger. 1990. Asian rickets and osteomalacia. *Quarterly Journal of Medicine* 76: 899–901.

Solomons, N. W., and R. A. Jacob. 1981. Studies on the bioavailability of zinc in humans: Effects of heme and non-heme iron on the absorption of zinc. *American Journal of Clinical Nutrition* 33: 739–45.

Sorensen, Ricardo U., Mary Catherine Porch, and Lan C. Tu. 1993. Food allergy in children. In Robert M. Suskind and Leslie Lewinter-Suskind, eds., *Textbook of Pediatric Nutrition,* 2nd ed. New York: Raven Press.

Sowers, MaryFran, Genie Corton, Brahm Shapiro, Mary L. Jannausch, Mary Crutchfield, Mindy L. Smith, John F. Randolph, and Bruce Hollis. 1993. Changes in bone density with lactation. *Journal of the American Medical Association* 269:24 (June 23/30): 3130–3135.

Soysa, Priyani. 1987. Women and nutrition. *World Review of Nutrition and Dietetics* 52: 1–70.

Specker, Bonnie L., Anne Black, Lindsay Allen, and Frank Morrow. 1990. Vitamin B_{12}: Low milk concentrations are related to low serum concentrations in vegetarian women and to methylmalonic aciduria in their infants. *American Journal of Clinical Nutrition* 52: 1073–76.

Spencer, Colin. 1993. *The Heretic's Feast: A History of Vegetarianism.* London: Fourth Estate.

Spencer, Herta, Lois Kramer, and Dace Osis. 1988. Do protein and phosphorus cause calcium loss? *Journal of Nutrition* 118: 657–60.

Srikantia, S. G., and V. Reddy. 1967. Megaloblastic anemia of infancy and vitamin B_{12}. *British Journal of Haematology* 13: 949–53.

Stevens, Richard G., Barry I. Graubard, Marc S. Micossi, Kazuo Neriishi, and Baruch
     S. Blumberg. 1994. Moderate elevation of body iron level and increased risk of
     cancer occurrence and death. *International Journal of Cancer* 56: 364–369.
Stollhoff, K., and F. J. Schulte. 1987. Vitamin B_{12} and brain development. *European
     Journal of Pediatrics* 146: 201–205.
Strause, Linda G., and Paul D. Saltman. 1993. Preventing bone loss with trace minerals
     and calcium supplementation. *Nutrition and the M.D.* 19:6 (June): 1–3.
Suskind, Robert M., and Leslie Lewinter-Suskind. 1993. *Textbook of Pediatric Nutrition*,
     2nd ed. New York: Raven Press.
Taliaferro, John, and Andrew Murr. 1991. National affairs: After police brutality: L.A.'s
     identity crisis. *Newsweek* 117:20 (May 20): 32–33.
Taub, Nadine, and Wendy W. Williams. 1985. Will equality require more than assimi-
     lation, accommodation, or separation from the existing social structure? *Rutgers
     Law Review/Civil Rights Developments* 37: 825 (reprinted in Smith 1993).
Taylor, Richard. 1991. *Virtue Ethics*. Interlaken, N.Y.: Linden Books.
Theophano, Janet, and Karen Curtis. 1991. Sisters, mothers, and daughters: Food
     exchange and reciprocity in an Italian-American community. In Anne Sharman,
     Janet Theophano, Karen Curtis, and Ellen Messer, eds., *Diet and Domestic Life in
     Society*, 147–72. Philadelphia: Temple University Press.
Tomasi, John. 1991. Individual ethics and community virtues. *Ethics* 101:3(April): 521–36.
Tong, Rosemarie. 1993. *Feminine and Feminist Ethics*. Belmont, Calif.: Wadsworth.
Trianosky, Gregory. 1990. What is virtue ethics all about? *American Philosophical Quar-
     terly* 27:4 (October): 335–344.
Truesdell, Delores D., and Phyllis B. Acosta. 1985. Feeding the vegan infant and child.
     Journal of the American Dietetic Association 85 (July): 837–40.
———, E. N. Whitney, and P. B. Acosta. 1984. Nutrients in vegetarian foods. *Journal
     of the American Dietetic Association* 84: 28–35.
Tuana, Nancy. 1993. *The Less Noble Sex: Scientific, Religious, and Philosophical Concep-
     tions of Woman's Nature*. Bloomington: Indiana University Press.
Tufts University. 1993. Warning: Keep dieting out of reach of children. *Tufts University
     Diet & Nutrition Letter* 11:10 (December): 3–6.
———. 1994a. Folic acid for fighting birth defects? *Tufts University Diet & Nutrition
     Letter* 10:9 (November): 1–2.
———. 1994b. Will the government take away your supplements? *Tufts University
     Diet & Nutrition Letter* 11:11 (January): 3–6.
Twigg, Julia. 1979. Food for thought: Purity and vegetarianism. *Religion* 9 (Spring): 13–35.
Tylavsky, Frances A., and John J. B. Anderson. 1988. Dietary factors in bone health of
     elderly lactoovovegetarian and omnivorous women. *American Journal of Clinical
     Nutrition* 48: 842–49.
United Nations. 1991. 1990 *Demographic Yearbook (Annuaire Demographique)*. New
     York: United Nations, Department of International Economic and Social Affairs,
     Statistical Office.
University of California. 1993. The new vegetarianism. *Berkeley Wellness Letter* 9:6
     (March): 4.

VanDeVeer, Donald. 1979. Interspecific justice. *Inquiry* 22:1–2 (Summer): 55–70.

Varner, Gary. 1994a. In defense of the vegan ideal. *Journal of Agricultural and Environmental Ethics* 7(1): 29–40.

———. 1994b. Rejoinder to Kathryn Paxton George. *Journal of Agricultural and Environmental Ethics* 7(1): 83–86.

———. 1994c. What's wrong with animal by-products? *Journal of Agricultural and Environmental Ethics* 7(1): 7–18.

Vlastos, Gregory. 1962. Justice and equality. In Richard B. Brandt, ed., *Social Justice*, 31–72. Englewood Cliffs, N.J.: Prentice-Hall.

Walker, Alice. 1983. *In Search of Our Mother's Gardens: Womanist Prose*. New York: Harcourt Brace Jovanovich.

Walkowitz, Judith R. 1982. Jack the Ripper and the myth of male violence. *Feminist Studies* 8: 543–574.

Wallace, James. 1978. *Virtues and Vices*. Ithaca, N.Y.: Cornell University Press.

Walravens, P. A., and K. M. Hambidge. 1976. Growth of infants fed a zinc supplemented formula. *American Journal of Clinical Nutrition* 29: 1114–21.

Walter, T., I. De Andraca, P. Chadud, and C. G. Perales. 1989. Iron deficiency anemia: Adverse effects on infant psychomotor development. *Pediatrics* 84: 7–17.

Wardlaw, Gordon M., and Paul M. Insel. 1993. *Perspectives in Nutrition*. 2nd ed. St. Louis: Mosby.

Warnock, Mary. 1962. Introduction. *John Stuart Mill, Utilitarianism, On Liberty, Essay on Bentham and Other Writings*. New York: New American Library.

Warren, Karen J. 1987. Feminism and ecology: Making connections. *Environmental Ethics* 9 (Spring): 3–20.

———. 1990. The power and promise of ecological feminism. *Environmental Ethics* 12:2 (Summer): 125–46.

———. 1993. Response to "Should feminists be vegetarians?" Paper presented at the Pacific Division meeting, American Philosophical Association, San Francisco, California, March 25, 1993.

Watson, James D. 1968. *The Double Helix: A Personal Account of the Discovery of the Structure of DNA*. New York: Atheneum.

Webb, A. R., L. Kline, and M. F. Holick. 1988. Influence of season and latitude on the cutaneous synthesis of vitamin D_3: Exposure to winter sunlight in Boston and Edmonton will not promote vitamin D_3 synthesis in human skin. *Journal of Clinical Endocrinology and Metabolism* 67: 373–378.

Whitbeck, Caroline. 1984. The maternal instinct. In Joyce Trebilcot, ed., *Mothering: Essays in Feminist Theory*. Totowa, N.J.: Rowman & Allanheld.

Whitney, Eleanor Noss and Eva May Nunnelley Hamilton. 1987. *Understanding Nutrition*. 4th ed. St. Paul: West Publishing Co.

Whorton, James C. 1994. Historical development of vegetarianism. *American Journal of Clinical Nutrition* 59 (supplement): 1103S–1109S.

Wighton, M.C., J. I. Manson, I. Speed, E. Robertson, and E. Chapman. 1979. Brain damage in infancy and dietary vitamin B_{12} deficiency. *Medical Journal of Australia* 2: 1–3.

Williams, A. J., and J. T. Ireland. 1977. Neonatal acidosis associated with transient methylmalonic aciduria and vitamin B_{12} deficiency. *Acta Paediatrica Scandinavica* 66: 117–19.

Wilson, Edward O. 1975. *Sociobiology: The New Synthesis.* Cambridge: Harvard University Press.

———. 1978. *On Human Nature.* Cambridge: Harvard University Press.

Wolf, Naomi. 1991. *The Beauty Myth: How Images of Beauty Are Used Against Women.* New York: William Morrow.

Wolgast, Elizabeth. 1980. *Equality and the Rights of Women.* Ithaca, N.Y.: Cornell University Press.

Wollstonecraft, Mary. 1792. *A Vindication of the Rights of Woman.* 2nd ed. London.

World Health Organization (WHO). 1987. Breastfeeding/breast milk and human immunodeficiency virus (HIV). *Weekly Epidemiological Record (Geneva)* 62: 245–46.

Wright, Robert. 1990. Are animals people too? *New Republic* (March 12): 20–22, 26–27.

Yokoi, Katsuhiko, and Harold H. Sandstead. 1992. Prospective overview [on the cause and prevention of Kak'ke. 1885. [Classical article by K. Takaki]. *Nutrition* 8:5 (September-October): 376–81.

Zhao, Xi-he. 1992. Nutritional situation of Beijing residents. *Southeast-Asian Journal of Tropical Medicine and Public Health* 23 (supplement 3): 65–68.

Zhu, H. 1990. Survey and analysis of incidence and relevant factors of osteoporosis in the elderly (with a report of 2041 cases). *Chung Hua I Hsueh Tsa Chih (Taipei)* 70: 5 (May): 248–51.

INDEX

absolutism: in Adams' view, 69; and paci-
    fism, 14–15; and rights, 28, 175 n. 9
absorption. *See* bioavailability
acceptance model, 137–39, 144–47
Adams, Carol J.: on animal rights, 5,
    67–70, 187 n. 2; appeals to purist
    ideals, 158–59, 188 n. 6; on use of
    animals, 142; use of feminist
    language, 188 n. 1; on veganism,
    113, 151, 159–60
allergies, food, 83, 101, 121–22
anemia: in developing countries, 94–95,
    113, 120; in pregnancy, 94–95; in
    United States, 94–95; with vitamin
    B$_{12}$ deficiency, 84–85, 100. *See also*
    iron, and vitamin B$_{12}$
animal(s): as differently situated, 140; and
    environment, 11, 13, 26;
    experimentation, 26; in feminine
    ethics of caring, 54; maltreatment
    of, 20; nature, 33, 139–40, 159;
    production, 13, 26; reasons for being
    unequal, 22; and right not to be
    killed, 27; rights, 4, 19, 61–62,
    67–70, 113; as "subjects-of-a-life,"
    5. *See also* factory farming
anorexia nervosa: definition of, 183 n. 31;
    and moral goodness, 109–12; as
    purity, 112; and zinc deficiency, 97
anti-cruelty view: defenses of, 27; defined,
    25; forbids inhumane treatment, 68;
    thinkers who reject, 25

anti-vivisectionism, 5, 49, 176 n. 3
arbitrariness:; of belief, 128; in ethics of
    care, 62; rejected by utilitarianism,
    34; ruled out by feminist ethics, 132
Aristotle: Doctrine of the Mean, 37;
    human nature, 32; list of virtues,
    40–41; virtue ethics, 35–39
assimilation model, 134–35, 140–42
autonomy: dialogical model of, 56;
    irreconcilable with femininity,
    111–12
availability. *See* bioavailability

Barbie doll, 109
beauty: and freedom, 108–09;
    intersubjective standard of, 156–57;
    and moral worth, 110, 183 n. 29
Bentham, Jeremy, 4, 26, 34, 175 n. 7
bias: personal, 124–26; reducing,
    122–24; in research studies,
    117–20
bioavailability: definition of, 88; heme-
    iron, 94; of iron in foods, 184 n. 4
body: affirmation of female, 127; animal,
    140; concept of, in dualism,
    158–59; as embodied spirit, 157;
    image disturbance, 92; unacceptable
    female, 108–09, 187 n. 1
bone: formation, 88–89, 100, 180 n. 12;
    health, 89–90; loss, 88–91, 104, 180
    n. 11
bulimia. *See* anorexia nervosa